Raj Chari and Isabel Rozas

Viruses, Vaccines, and Antivirals: Why Politics Matters

Viral Politics

Volume 1

Raj Chari and Isabel Rozas

Viruses, Vaccines, and Antivirals: Why Politics Matters

—

DE GRUYTER

ISBN (Paperback) 978-3-11-076484-0
ISBN (Hardcover) 978-3-11-074358-6
e-ISBN (PDF) 978-3-11-074360-9
e-ISBN (EPUB) 978-3-11-074372-2
ISSN 2747-6863
e-ISSN 2747-6871

Library of Congress Control Number: 2021943984

Bibliographic information published by the Deutsche Nationalbibliothek
The Deutsche Nationalbibliothek lists this publication in the Deutsche Nationalbibliografie;
detailed bibliographic data are available on the Internet at http://dnb.dnb.de.

© 2022 Walter de Gruyter GmbH, Berlin/Boston
Cover image: CROCOTHERY / iStock / Getty Images Plus
Printing and binding: CPI books GmbH, Leck

www.degruyter.com

For Celia Chari Rozas

Acknowledgements

This book would not have been possible without the excellent research assistance performed by an amazing group of young scholars who form part of the Viral-Politics project (www.viral-politics.com): Clare Elwell, Laura Grindle, Xenia Kadar, Daire McCutcheon, Jack O'Neill, Alannah Owens, Adeyemi Rahman, Lily Rice, and Liam Smith.

We are indebted to Tony Mason, Gerhard Boomgaarden, Michaela Göbels and all the team in De Gruyter for their insights, enthusiasm and encouragement. We are also grateful to the three anonymous reviewers for their excellent suggestions.

Finally, we thank José Elguero for fantastic observations and Arlene Healy for kindly ensuring access to resources through the Library at Trinity College Dublin.

RC & IR, Dublin, July 2021

https://doi.org/10.1515/9783110743609-001

Contents

List of figures

List of graphs

Chapter 1
Introduction

On January 7, 2020 the SARS-CoV-2 coronavirus was identified in workers of the 'wet market' in Wuhan as the infective agent responsible for the unusual pneumonias detected since December 2019. This was only the beginning of one of the most uncertain periods for humanity since the Second World War: the COVID-19 pandemic.

On that date, there was no indication that the virus was spreading easily because some infected people were asymptomatic. Soon, the infection had moved to nearby countries such as Thailand, South Korea and Japan. Before it was contained, it had already spread as far as the US, Australia, Italy and Spain. The World Health Organization (WHO), previously accused of being alarmist when dealing with the 2003 SARS coronavirus outbreak, cautiously declared this viral infection a Public Health Emergency of International Concern on January 30, 2020. Soon after, all around the world, cities became empty while people died alone in hospitals and, beyond the human tragedy, the global economy suffered a tremendous blow.

Despite earnest criticisms made against many governments and international institutions, nobody saw this coming and nobody was ready for it. For that reason, this book aims to give guidance to governments to be ready for future pandemics, since this is neither the first one, nor will it be the last. Based on natural science concepts around viruses, viral infection prevention (i.e. vaccines) and antiviral treatments, and considering the different stages of the pandemic seen in different countries, we propose a typology that can serve as a blueprint for states to deal with future health crises.

Thus, in Chapter 2 we offer an overview of the 'natural science' side of our investigation by first considering what a virus is and outlining key terms and nomenclature. We then examine previous pandemics, including the plague, smallpox, malaria, cholera, tuberculosis, and AIDS. Next, we turn to the present pandemic, focusing on coronaviruses, viral replication, COVID-19 and SARS-CoV-2 variants. In the rest of the chapter, attention is then paid to putting a drug on the market, antiviral therapies to treat COVID-19, and vaccines to prevent it.

Given the importance of governments in developing public policies when there is no immediate anti-viral treatment or vaccine during a pandemic, the public policies they formulate are paramount. Hence, Chapter 3 starts with the 'social science' side of our research by first looking at the historical role of the state during pandemics. We then explain why over time the WHO has not been pivotal in shaping how countries have responded. This has resulted in

https://doi.org/10.1515/9783110743609-002

states largely 'going it alone' and rather blindly developing public policy responses, which was particularly evident during COVID-19. The second part of the chapter thus develops a typology of four phases of policy responses to guide states during a pandemic: anticipating the virus, containing it, controlling it, and then opening up society. Here we outline the empirical indicators that signal the start of the phases and the policies that are expected to be found in each of the phases. The strength of our classification scheme is that it can be used to understand developments in any country, anytime, during any pandemic.

Next, Chapter 4 demonstrates the strength of this typology by examining public policies pursued in key countries during the COVID-19 pandemic against the expectations in our typology. In the first part of the chapter we justify the countries examined and explain the mixed methods approach relying on both qualitative and quantitative methodologies used for our country analysis. We then examine developments in these countries as follows: New Zealand, Ireland, Germany, Canada, the United States, India, South Africa and Chile. The chapter closes with comparative examination of the COVID-19 vaccination rollout in these states.

Finally, Chapter 5 closes by highlighting the main findings of the book. It also outlines significant lessons to be taken from this study, from both the 'natural science' and 'social science' vantages.

It is our overall objective that this book represents an incremental, as opposed to a step, change in scholarship because it examines a key global crisis in the last century for a broad group of readers. Those interested in social science will better understand the science behind viral infections, how to treat and prevent them, and why evidence-based policy is important when evaluating policymakers' decisions. Those more oriented towards natural science and medicine will better understand what governments are doing (or not doing) to deal with health crises. While there are many books and papers on COVID-19, we believe that this book represents a novel attempt to fruitfully bring both the natural and social scientific communities together, serving as a strong foundation for more interdisciplinary research.

Chapter 2
Viruses, antivirals and vaccines

In this chapter we offer an essential overview of viruses, pandemics, vaccines, and antiviral treatments and development, situating the importance of this in contextualizing political decisions. Our view is that while the world has watched what has happened during the COVID-19 crisis, there is a lack of information on the basic facts about the 'science' side. Examining this will be particularly useful for social scientists seeking to situate where governments find themselves during any viral pandemic.

So ... What is a virus?

Viruses are not animals or plants, and they are also different to bacteria; however, they are the most amazing parasites. They are the simplest entities and their existence as 'living' beings has been questioned. Basic requisites for an entity to be considered 'alive' are to be able to reproduce by itself, to move by itself and to store energy (adenosine triphosphate – ATP – in biological terms). Viruses do not comply with any of these requisites; they need an animal or plant cell, the *host*, to reproduce themselves, they do not store any ATP, and they are entirely dependent on external physical factors for movement and propagation. They also parasitize the cell to obtain basic materials such as amino acids and nucleotides, which are needed to build more viruses. Without a host, viruses cannot exist.

The structure of a virus is fascinating. Viruses consist exclusively of two types of macromolecules: nucleic acids (deoxyribonucleic acid – DNA – or ribonucleic acid – RNA) and proteins (Figure 2.1).

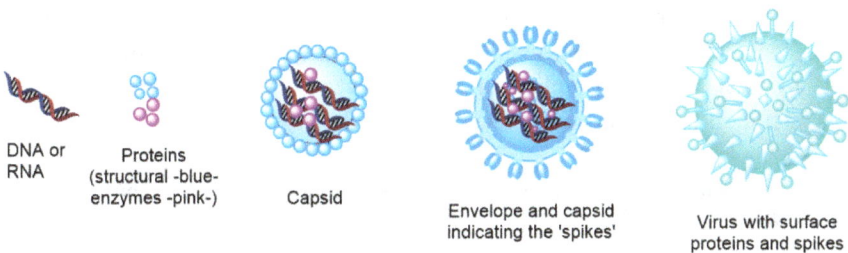

DNA or RNA

Proteins (structural -blue- enzymes -pink-)

Capsid

Envelope and capsid indicating the 'spikes'

Virus with surface proteins and spikes

Figure 2.1: Schematic representation of the elements comprising a virus and how they form the viral structure.

https://doi.org/10.1515/9783110743609-003

Nucleic acids store all genetic information, the genome, which contains all the 'instructions' to build future viruses. Proteins can play two different roles, surround and protect the genome (structural proteins) or help with the viral reproduction (enzymes). The core of a virus is formed by the corresponding nucleic acid (DNA or RNA, but never both) closely folded and tightly covered by a layer of protein units (capsomers) that form the '(nucleo)capsid' to protect the viral genome (Figure 2.1).

Curiously, these capsids can adopt icosahedral or helical shapes. Many viruses have also a roughly spherical lipidic 'envelope' that protects the capsid. Embedded in the capsid or in the envelope there are other types of proteins (glycoproteins), known as 'spikes', that help the virus to attach to the host cells (Figure 2.2).

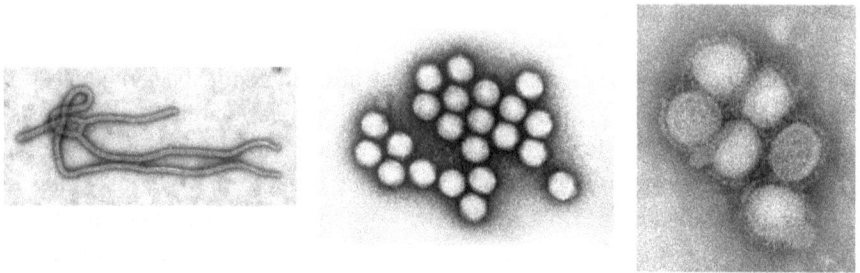

Figure 2.2: Microscope images of three examples of viruses with different capsids' structures, from left to right, helical (Ebola – CDC/ Cynthia Goldsmith, Courtesy: Public Health Image Library), icosahedral (adenovirus – CDC/ Dr. G. William Gary, Jr., Courtesy: Public Health Image Library) and enveloped (influenza – CDC/ C. S. Goldsmith and A. Balish, Courtesy: Public Health Image Library).

The most common virus classification system is the Baltimore classification (Figure 2.3) which groups viruses into seven families depending on
(i)   the type of nucleic acid (DNA or RNA) that they contain,
(ii) number of strands of the nucleic acid: double-stranded (ds) DNA or RNA or single-stranded (ss) RNA with a positive or negative 'sense', and
(iii) by their method of replication (i.e. retroviruses that require reverse transcription to DNA before replication can take place).

Some examples of viruses belonging to the different families in the Baltimore classification are human herpes virus (class I), parvovirus (class II), rotavirus – childhood gastroenteritis (class III), coronavirus (class IV), Ebola virus (class V), human immunodeficiency virus (class VI), hepatitis B (class VII).

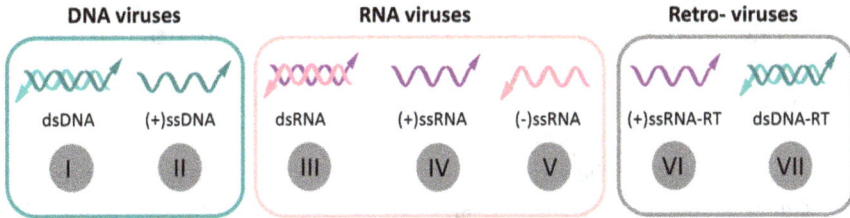

Figure 2.3: Baltimore classification of viruses based on their nucleic acid (DNA or RNA), single or double strand (ss or ds) and positive or negative sense single strand.

As mentioned, coronaviruses (CoV) belong to class IV, which includes single stranded RNA viruses with a positive sense strand (represented by the notation (+)ssRNA) such as picornavirus (e. g. hepatitis A), togavirus/matonavirus (e. g. rubella) or flavivirus (e. g. zika). There are several viruses that belong to the CoV family, but those that have raised more concern to humans in the recent years are

- the 'severe acute respiratory syndrome coronavirus' (SARS-CoV) which caused an epidemic in 2002–03,
- the 'Middle East respiratory syndrome-related coronavirus' (MERS-CoV) that became a threat in 2012 and
- the 'severe acute respiratory syndrome coronavirus 2' (SARS-CoV-2), which is the cause of the present 2019–20 COVID-19 'pandemic'.

A bit of nomenclature

Before going ahead with this chapter, several terms need to be clearly defined. According to the Principles of Epidemiology in Public Health Practice an '*epidemic* refers to an increase, often sudden, in the number of cases of a disease above what is normally expected in that population in that area' while '*pandemic* refers to an epidemic that has spread over several countries or continents, usually affecting a large number of people.'[1] Other related terms, that will be used in the following chapters, are *outbreak* that is defined as an epidemic in 'a more limited geographic area' and *cluster* that 'refers to an aggregation of cases grouped in place and time that are suspected to be greater than the number expected.'[2]

---

1 https://www.cdc.gov/csels/dsepd/ss1978/lesson1/section11.html
2 Ibid.

At the beginning of the present pandemic there was an extensive discussion on the origin of the viral infection and the term *zoonotic* appeared in the news. Thus, *zoonotic* refers to the spread of germs between animals and people due to daily interactions of humans with animals at work or at home.

Throughout this chapter we will be talking about the spread of the infection that occurs because of the viral replication cycle involving the *transcription* and *translation* of the viral genome. Thus, we will explain how once inside the host cell, SARS-CoV-2 takes over the host machinery to *transcribe* and *translate* its (+) ss-RNA genome into structural and functional proteins before the new viruses are assembled, encapsulated, and budded out of the cell. This will be discussed in detail later on in this chapter and here we will only explain what the terms *transcription* and *translation* mean. The process of *transcription* consists of transforming the viral genome into messenger RNA (mRNA) and this is performed by enzymes named polymerases, whereas translation consists of producing proteins based on the information provided by the mRNA and making use of another nucleic acid, the transfer RNA or tRNA (Figure 2.4).

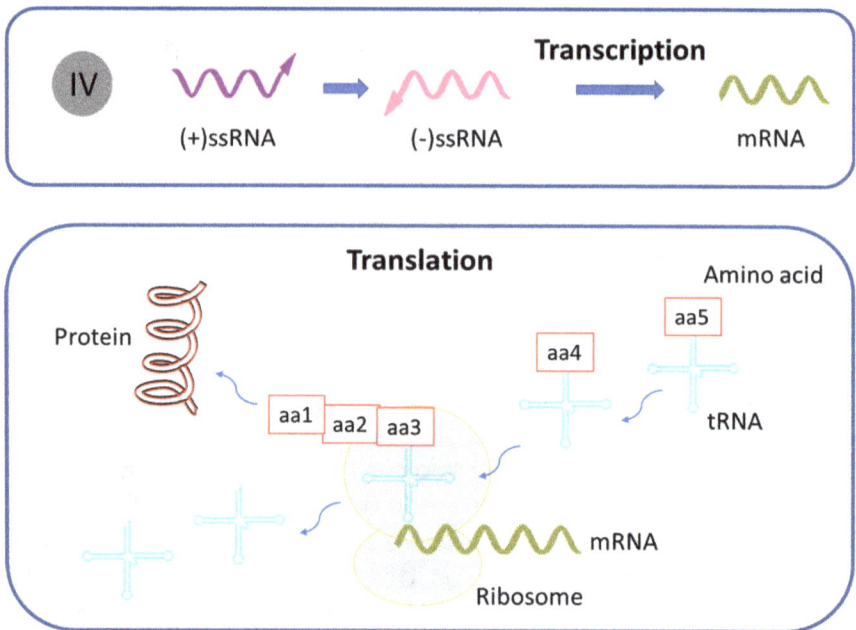

Figure 2.4: Scheme of the processes of *transcription*, which is the production of the messenger RNA (mRNA) in the case of class IV viruses (i. e. containing (+)ssRNA) and *translation*, which is the transformation of the genetic information of mRNA into amino acids carried by the transfer RNA (tRNA) to form the corresponding protein.

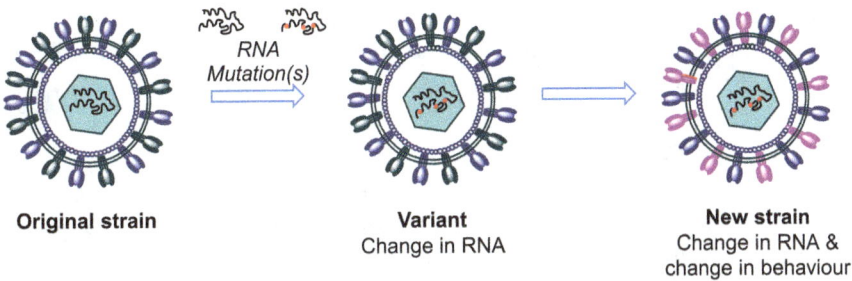

Original strain	Variant	New strain
	RNA Mutation(s)	
	Change in RNA	Change in RNA & change in behaviour

Figure 2.5: Viruses with mutations become variants and when variants show different properties to the original virus, they are named a new strain.

Recently, the appearance of *variants* has increased the number of cases and severity of the pandemic. It is important then to define what a *mutation* is and to distinguish between *variants* and *strains* (Figure 2.5). A *mutation* is defined as the changing of the structure of a gene (DNA or RNA) in the reproductive step and results from an error in the replication of that particular nucleic acid (Figure 2.5). After translation of the gene to produce the corresponding proteins, this change produces a modification in the resulting protein. Thus, mutations are usually identified by a letter, a number, and another letter, where the first letter represents the amino acid in the position indicated by the 'number' (starting from the N-terminal) of the original protein and the last letter represents the new amino acid that appears in that position as a consequence of the gene mutation. Thus, the E484K mutation (important in many SARS-CoV-2 variants) indicates the substitution of a glutamic acid (E), that was in the position 484 of the original spike protein, by a lysine (K) in the mutated protein.

When a virus multiplies by making copies of itself, it sometimes makes small mistakes that are called mutations, and a virus with a small number of mutations is called a *variant* of the original virus. However, when there is such a large number of mutations that makes the *variant* virus behave differently to the original one, it is called a new *strain*. Essentially, all strains are variants, but not all variants are strains.

We will discuss viral detection tests based on identifying *antigens* or *antibodies* later. *Antigens* are proteins present in the virus that can trigger an immune response in the body, since they are identified as 'foreign' molecules that can be dangerous for the body. *Antibodies* are the molecules produced by the body as a response to an infection; they are produced when an *antigen* is identified by the immune system.

Additionally, it should be clarified that SARS-CoV-2 is the name given to the virus, while COVID-19 (COrona VIrus Disease of 2019) is what the disease has been called; this is similar to the case of AIDS (Acquired ImmunoDeficiency Syndrome), which is the disease caused by the Human Immunodeficiency Virus (HIV).

Previous pandemics

As mentioned, *pandemic* refers to an infection affecting a large number of people. These infections can be produced by different microorganisms such as bacteria or viruses. The world has seen several *pandemics* and some of the most important to mention are the plague, smallpox, malaria, cholera, tuberculosis, influenza and AIDS.

Probably the oldest known pandemic is the plague, which is an infectious disease produced by a bacterium, *Yersinia pestis*, that can be found in small mammals and their fleas. Hence, this is a *zoonotic* bacterium since it can be transmitted from animals to humans by the bite of infected fleas. Plague can be very severe in human beings, producing septicaemia or pneumonia, and with a case/fatality ratio between 30 and 100 % if left untreated. Throughout history, there have been up to three major plague pandemics, with that of 1347 (i.e. Black Death) being the most lethal since it decimated half of the European continent's population. However, today this infection can be easily treated with antibiotics and some preventive standard measures. Plague is still found worldwide (except Oceania), but the Democratic Republic of Congo, Madagascar and Peru are the most endemic countries. According to the WHO, 'to prevent the plague, inactivated bacterial vaccines have been used since 1890'; however, over time 'more effective live, attenuated vaccines and recombination protein vaccines have been developed... to prevent the disease.'[3]

The smallpox pandemic caused by the variola virus was devastating, causing millions of deaths for more than 3000 years until a vaccine was found and it was finally declared eradicated in 1980.[4] The story of the development of this vaccine is quite interesting and involves several women whose names have been forgotten. We know that inoculation of the pus of blisters from smallpox infected cows was known to have been used in China since the X century to prevent the disease. Much later, around the beginning of the XVIII century a British aristocrat, Lady Mary Montagu, when traveling in Turkey realized that local people practised inoculation against smallpox (i.e. variolation) by introducing pus taken from a mild smallpox blister into scratched skin, and even though

---

3 https://www.who.int/health-topics/plague#tab=tab_1
4 https://www.who.int/health-topics/smallpox#tab=tab_1

they developed a mild case of the disease they never suffered the serious condition. Therefore, she decided to inoculate her 5-year-old son and when she was back in England she was able to disseminate the procedure to other people, including some children in the royal family.[5] Despite this success, the medical establishment strongly opposed the method and it was not until a man, Edward Jenner, developed the vaccine 90 years later, that this procedure was understood. Jenner realized that milkmaids who got cowpox (a mild version of smallpox) did not develop the serious disease and then he reckoned that by inoculating this mild version smallpox could be prevented in people (Riedel, 2005). Another woman that contributed to this type of inoculation against smallpox was the Spanish nurse Isabel Zendal who at the beginning of the XIX century took part in the three-year Balmis expedition which brought the smallpox vaccination to South America. She had been overseeing an orphanage in Galicia (the northwest of Spain) and her role in the expedition was to take care of 26 orphan boys who carried the mild version of the virus from which the vaccine was prepared.[6] In 1967, the WHO launched a plan to eradicate smallpox by conducting widespread immunization and surveillance around the world, and in 1980 smallpox was declared eradicated by the WHO.

Malaria is a severe disease transmitted to humans by the bites of female Anopheles mosquitoes infected by *Plasmodium* parasites. From all the parasite species that cause malaria in humans, *P. falciparum* and *P. vivax* represent the greatest threat. Despite being a preventable and curable disease, in 2019 there were around 229 million cases worldwide, where the African region experienced the highest burden (i.e. 94% of cases and deaths) followed by other regions at risk such as South-East Asia, Eastern Mediterranean, Western Pacific, and the Americas.[7] There is now a battery of antimalarial drugs to prevent and treat malaria. Thus, in the case of pregnant women and children, the WHO recommends no less than three doses of preventive treatment with sulfadoxine-pyrimethamine intermittently. Since 2012, as an additional strategy, the WHO recommends preventive seasonal malaria treatments for some areas in Africa. Only one vaccine, 'RTS,S', has been developed so far and it significantly reduces malaria (even the most severe form) in children by acting against *P. falciparum*. This vaccine seems to be able to prevent 4 in 10 cases and lasts for four years. Additionally, controlling the 'vectors' (i.e. mosquitoes) is an effective measure of protection against malaria and some examples of these vector control methods are

---

5 https://time.com/5542895/mary-montagu-smallpox/
6 https://www.mujeresenlahistoria.com/2015/08/la-dama-de-la-vacuna-isabel-zendal-1773.html
7 https://www.who.int/news-room/fact-sheets/detail/malaria

insecticide-treated nets and indoor spraying. According to McMillen (2016, 45), control of the malaria pandemic was 'tied to the goal of fostering democracy and capitalism and stemming the tide of communism'. The argument made in 1956 by the US International Development Administration was that controlling malaria would ease urban overcrowding in the regions of Java, Vietnam and the Philippines, and that allowing DDT spraying in those areas would facilitate landless peasants to become successful farmers. In this way they foresaw the control of malaria as a way to control communism and spread capitalist democracy. Political spin aside, in the last 20 years eleven countries have been certified by the WHO as malaria-free: United Arab Emirates (2007), Morocco (2010), Turkmenistan (2010), Armenia (2011), Sri Lanka (2016), Kyrgyzstan (2016), Paraguay (2018), Uzbekistan (2018), Algeria (2019), Argentina (2019) and El Salvador (2021), and in January 2021 the WHO published extended guidance for countries for a sustained elimination.[8]

Despite the general perception that cholera is a disease of the past, the reality that it is still prevalent in underdeveloped countries, and a pandemic has been ongoing since 1961. Cholera is produced when *Vibrio cholerae* bacteria infect the small intestine. The disease, which affects around 2.9 million people and causes around 95,000 deaths per year, is endemic in more than 47 countries worldwide. Factors such as climate change, long war conflicts, population growth, and more importantly poor access to health facilities are associated with cholera outbreaks. This infection could be prevented by the Oral Cholera Vaccine and can be easily treated with oral rehydration solution; however, since this disease is acquired by ingesting contaminated water, it could be more efficiently prevented by an appropriate investment in suitable water and sanitation infrastructure.[9]

Tuberculosis, which is a very infectious bacterial infection (i.e. only a few germs inhaled are enough to become infected), is also an on-going pandemic. TB, as it is commonly referred to, results from infection by the bacteria *Mycobacterium tuberculosis*, which was discovered by Robert Koch in 1882. A genetic study in 2014 (Bos et al., 2014) suggested that the most recent common ancestor dates from only 6000 years ago; however, there is evidence that the first TB infection occurred around 9000 years ago (Hershkovitz et al., 2008) and it has been proposed that this infection spread to domestic and wild animals in Africa with seals exporting it to South America (Bos et al., 2014). TB, which is spread through the air by an infected person coughing or sneezing can be preventable;

---

8 https://www.who.int/health-topics/malaria#tab=tab_1
9 https://www.who.int/health-topics/cholera#tab=tab_1

however, 10 million people fall ill with TB every year and around 1.5 million people die.[10] Antibiotics can cure TB infections, but resistance has developed making this condition a problem, mostly among HIV patients. Considering that both *M. tuberculosis* and SARS-CoV-2 affect primarily the lungs, there is concern that TB patients contracting COVID-19 could have very poor treatment outcomes. Despite the development of a vaccine at the beginning of the XX century (BCG vaccine), it has not been very successful and nowadays only a few countries use it routinely.

Influenza's more famous pandemic happened between 1918 and 1919. It was caused by the H1N1 influenza A virus and it is estimated to have killed between 50 and 100 million people. Even though the first observations of this pandemic were located in the US, France, Germany and the UK, this information was censored in the corresponding countries due to the on-going World War I. However, in Spain, which was a neutral country, information about the pandemic was freely reported, including the fact that it had affected the king himself. This gave the impression that Spain had been in the origin of the pandemic and for that reason it was wrongly denominated 'Spanish Flu'.[11] The most recent influenza pandemics are those known as bird-flu (between 2007–08, caused by H5N1 strand) and swine-flu (2009, caused by the H1N1 strand). There are four different influenza viruses: the A type affects humans and pigs among other mammals, types B and C mostly affect humans, and the D type infects mostly cattle and pigs. Types A and B are responsible for seasonal flu epidemics while the C type causes a mild infection usually in children. Influenza viruses are transmitted through coughing and sneezing as well as aerosols (i.e. very small droplets containing the virus). The influenza viruses mutate rapidly, and it is for that reason that there is a need for annual vaccination to deal with the corresponding strain of that particular year. Current vaccines protect mostly against the H1N1 and H3N2 strains of type A.[12]

Probably one of the best-known pandemics nowadays, before the present COVID-19, is that resulting from HIV infection (AIDS), which has now killed around 30 million and infected 75 million people worldwide (McMillen, 2016, 104). The epidemic emergence of HIV in the late XIX – early XX century and the lack of previous emergences can be explained by increasing human exposures to Simian Immunodeficiency Virus (SIV). Thus, the growth of cities in the 1880s in Central Africa probably played a role in the HIV epidemic emergence

---

10 https://www.who.int/health-topics/tuberculosis#tab=tab_1
11 https://theconversation.com/10-misconceptions-about-the-1918-flu-the-greatest-pandemic-in-history-133994
12 https://www.atrainceu.com/content/2-influenza-virus-types-and-subtypes-0

because the phylogenetic dating of the oldest strains of HIV suggests that they started to spread shortly after the main Central African colonial cities were founded. HIV infections may have emerged because of colonialism, particularly in Belgian Equatorial Africa, where workers were submitted to severe conditions, displacement, and forced labour, and were provided with bushmeat for food, thus exposing them to SIV. The colonial authorities also vaccinated workers against smallpox, using unsafe or unsterile injections between uses. Finally, the prostitution associated with forced labour camps could have caused serial transmission of SIV between humans helped by genital ulcer diseases (i. e. syphilis, chancroid, or genital herpes), since these provide a portal of viral entry. All this was reflected in Joseph Conrad's book, *Heart of Darkness,* where he describes the life of an ivory transporter down the Congo River in Central Africa and also in the novel *The Dream of the Celt* by Mario Vargas Llosa, which depicts the life of the Irishman Roger Casement in Congo. Development of antiretroviral therapies (ARTs) have resulted in a serious decrease of AIDS related deaths and the use of prevention measures (i. e. condoms, one-use syringes, among others) has also diminished the number of new infections. Additionally, ARTs are being used as prophylaxis treatments for pre- (PrEP) or post- (PEP) exposure to the virus, and this also has had an enormous impact in the life of couples where one is HIV positive and the other negative as well as for health workers that accidentally get infected.[13] Even though many research efforts have been devoted to the development of a HIV vaccine, this has not yet been achieved. Some reasons for this failure so far can be the high level of mutability of this virus; that attenuated viruses used for the development of vaccines are still dangerous to humans; or the lack of reliable animal models to test the vaccine.

Present pandemic: coronaviruses, viral replication and SARS-CoV-2 variants

The present COVID-19 pandemic is not the first one caused by a coronavirus. In fact, previous outbreaks of coronavirus infection were a global threat in 2002–03 (by the Severe Acute Respiratory Syndrome, SARS) and in 2011 (by Middle East Respiratory Syndrome, MERS). In both pandemics, the causative viruses (SARS-CoV and MERS-CoV) were identified as new coronaviruses.

Coronaviruses can produce 'a variety of diseases in mammals and birds ranging from enteritis in cows and pigs and upper respiratory disease in chick-

---

13 https://www.cdc.gov/hiv/clinicians/prevention/prep-and-pep.html

ens to potentially lethal human respiratory infections' (Fehr and Perlman, 2015, 1). These viruses have an spherical shape with a diameter around 125 nm, contain an unusually large RNA genome, and their characteristic club-shape spikes (S) emanating from the surface of the virus give them the appearance of a solar corona; hence, their name (Figure 2.6).

While the origin of these CoV infections is still not fully confirmed, possible transmission from animals (zoonotic transmission) may be considered. This is not unusual for viruses in general. In fact, as mentioned the HIV, causative of AIDS, is a good example since its connection to the SIV is well established. Therefore, it is quite plausible that coronaviruses have been transmitted from animals. In the case of MERS, it seems clear that the zoonotic transmission took place from infected camels that could have been infected by bats, whereas in the case of SARS the transmission to humans seems to have arisen from the manipulation of the meat of pangolins that had been infected by bats. In the present pandemic produced by the SARS-Cov-2, the animal species that may be responsible for the zoonotic transmission is still unclear, but considering that coronaviruses are known to infect bats these animals have been proposed as potential zoonotic origin (Andersen et al., 2020; Zhou P et al., 2020).

In more detail, in May 2020 the WHO organized a working group 'to identify the zoonotic source of the virus and the route of introduction to the human pop-

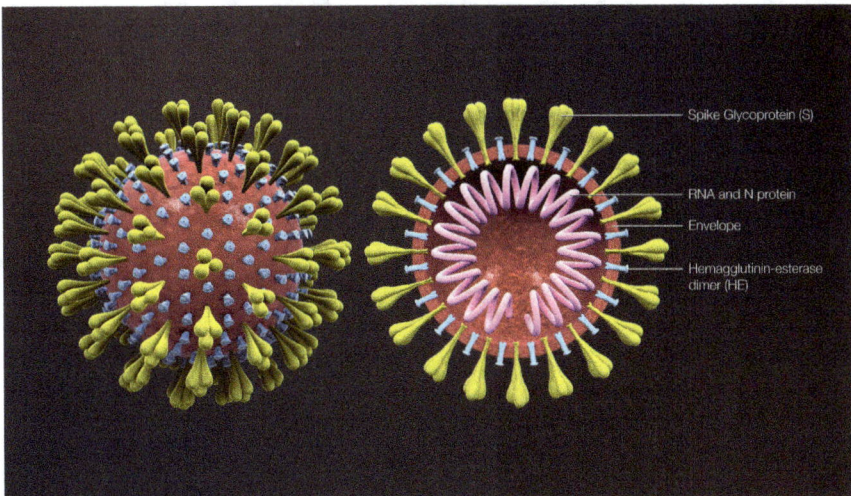

Figure 2.6: Structure of a corona virus indicating the spike glycoprotein, the nucleic acid (RNA), different viral enzymes and the envelope. Image created by https://www.scientificani mations.com – https://www.scientificanimations.com/wiki-images/, CC BY-SA 4.0, https://com mons.wikimedia.org/w/index.php?curid=86358105

ulation' in order to 'prevent both reinfection with the virus in animals and humans and the establishment of new zoonotic reservoirs, thereby reducing further risks of the emergence and transmission of zoonotic diseases' (WHO, 2021, 6). In the first stage of this study, they concluded that the SARS-CoV-2 isolated from humans were genetically related to coronaviruses found in bats. They also stated that considering the similarity in the SARS-CoV-2 genetic sequences so far isolated from humans, it is likely that the origin of the outbreak came from a single point around the time that the first case in humans was reported in Wuhan (China) and that the spread from animal to humans occurred during the last months of 2019. In February 2021, a team of WHO experts spent four weeks in Wuhan to research this further and concluded that '(t)he findings suggest lab incident hypothesis is extremely unlikely to explain the introduction of the virus into the human population,' that SARS-CoV-2 'may have originated from zoonotic transmission', but the 'reservoir hosts' need still to be identified.[14] These experts did not find evidence that there had been large outbreaks before December 2019. They recommended to continue examining the direct spread from animals to humans and further research frozen foods as potential intermediates in the transmission; however, they could not find any indication of the role of the Huanan Seafood Wholesale Market in the origin of the infection because they found cases related to this market as well as unrelated cases (WHO, 2021).

The process of infection of a virus to the human cells (host), known as the 'replication cycle', involves several steps leading to the production of new viruses (virions) and the amplification of the infection. In the case of SARS-CoV-2, which as mentioned is a (+)ss-RNA coronavirus, the cycle starts with the attachment and entry of the virus into the human host cell. This step occurs by means of the attachment of the S protein present in the viral spikes to the angiotensin-converting enzyme 2 (ACE2) receptor expressed in the surface of lungs, arteries, heart, kidneys, and intestine cells (Zhou F et al., 2020). More specifically, the S protein is cleaved into two subunits (S1 and S2) and while S1 binds to ACE2, S2 is activated by another host surface enzyme, the transmembrane protease serine 2 (TMPRSS2) (Hoffman et al., 2020a). Interaction of the viral spike with both the ACE2 receptor and the TMPRSS2 protease results in the fusion of the membranes of host and virus, driving to the entry of the virus in the human host, and then releasing the RNA genome into the cytoplasm (Figure 2.7).

Next, the virus takes over the host translation machinery and thus the cell will translate the viral messenger RNA (mRNA) into structural proteins and enzymes for the new virions instead of producing proteins for the host. These

---

14 https://www.irishexaminer.com/world/arid-40223153.html

newly translated viral proteins recruit the RNA into a membrane of the endoplasmic reticulum (cell organelle) to form the replication complex together with an enzyme (i.e. RNA-dependent RNA polymerase), in order to synthesize a negative (-)ss-RNA (Liu et al., 2020; Fehr and Perlman, 2015). This replication complex is then used as a template to transcribe and replicate the complete viral RNA genome in several copies, thus amplifying the viral (+)ss-RNA. Next, the newly synthesized viral proteins and RNA copies are transferred from the endoplasmic reticulum through the Golgi apparatus (cell organelles), where new viruses assemble (Fehr and Perlman, 2015). Finally, the mature SARS-CoV-2 viruses are exocytosed and released from the host cell where the infection cycle will repeat several times (Guo et al., 2020) (Figure 2.7).

To continue spreading, SARS-CoV-2 is evolving to evade the human immune system. Thus, several variants of SARS-CoV-2 have been identified around the world so far such as the Californian B1.427/9, New York B.1.526, Nigerian B.1.1.207, and Belgian B.1.214, each containing different mutations. However, the most extended have been the Spanish variant (B.1.177), the UK variant (B.1.1.7, now named *alpha* by the WHO), the South African variant (B.1.351, now named *beta*), the Brazilian variant (P.1, now named *gamma*) and, more recently, the Indian variant (B.1.617.2, now named *delta*).[15]

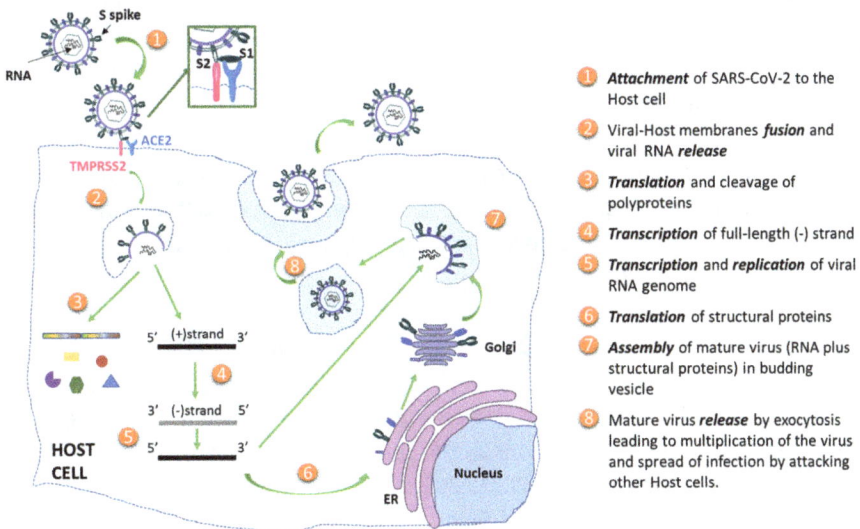

Figure 2.7: Infection/replication cycle of SARS-CoV-2 into a lung host cell.

---

15 https://www.who.int/en/activities/tracking-SARS-CoV-2-variants/

The Spanish variant (B.1.177 or 20E(EU1)) was most extensive in the EU since the summer 2020 and it results from one specific mutation (S477N) in an area of the spike protein of the virus not directly involved in the entry to the host cells (Tortorici et al., 2020; McCallum et al., 2020; Walls et al., 2020). In a collaborative study carried out between the US, Switzerland and Spain, it was found that this variant did not increase transmissibility; hence, the high incidence found was due to the resumption of traveling across the EU and the failure in the screening and quarantine policies (Hodcroft et al., 2021). The case of the UK variant (*alpha*) is different since it shows a very high level of transmission; this B.1.1.7 variant started to spread worldwide in Q4 of 2020 and shows a large number of mutations (e. g. N501Y, 69 – 70del, P681H) mostly in the spike protein. In particular, the N501Y mutation seems to facilitate the binding of the viral spike to the host receptor ACE2 which is the point of entry of the SARS-CoV-2 virus into several human cells as explained before. In a recent study (Davies et al., 2021) it has been estimated that the *alpha*-variant is not only more transmissible than previously known variants, but also more lethal since the risk of death is around 61 % higher because it causes a more severe disease. The *beta* variant (B.1.351) appeared around October 2020 independently of the B.1.1.7. This B.1.351 variant shows several mutations (i. e. N501Y, K417N, E484K), few common to those in the *alpha* variant. The *beta* variant can reinfect people who have recovered from other variants. The *gamma* variant (P.1) seems to have appeared around December 2020 with some mutations similar to the B.1.1.7 and B.1.351 variants (i. e. N501Y, E484K, K417T). It was identified first in people traveling from Brazil to Japan and South Korea. Mortality associated with this variant may be higher than that of the *alpha* or *beta* variants. The E484K mutation, which is common to the *beta* and *gamma* variants, occurs in the spike protein and may be responsible for stopping the antibodies from neutralizing the virus, thus reducing the effectiveness of the AstraZeneca and Moderna vaccines (Weisblum et al., 2020). According to the CDC, all these three variants share the D614G specific mutation that allows the virus to spread faster.

The large number of cases observed in the second wave of SARS-CoV-2 infection in India are the result of the new *delta* variant (B.1.617), which appeared in a region of India (Maharashtra) in February 2021. The rapid increase in cases could be the result of specific mutations in the spike protein and significant co-occurring 'triple mutations' (i. e. L452R, E484Q and P681); for this reason this variant is wrongly referred to as the 'triple mutation' variant, even though up to 15 mutations have been detected.[16] Genome analysis of B.1.617 indicates that it ap-

---

16 https://www.newscientist.com/definition/indian-covid-19-variant-b-1-617/ and https://www.

peared independently in India and is quite different to the *alpha, beta* or *gamma* variants since all the 15 mutations observed are dissimilar to those found in the other variants with the exception of L452R (found also in the California variant B.1.427/429) and E484K (found also in the B.1.351, P.1, and B.1.526 variants). Mutations at the 484 position have been observed in many variants of the SARS-CoV-2 virus, but in the particular case of the *delta* variant the amino acid change occurring at this position is different with a E484Q mutation being observed.

We now consider some of the most relevant mutations found in the current variants, which are responsible for the large surges, faster spread and more casualties as seen in late 2020 and early 2021. One of the most common mutations in all SARS-CoV-2 variants is the D614G, where the Aspartic acid (D) at position 614 of the spike protein of the virus has been replaced by a Glycine (G). The prevalence of this mutation seems to indicate that it is the cause behind higher rates of transmission. Another very common mutation found in the *beta* and *gamma* variants is the E484K (a Glutamic acid E in position 484 is replaced by a Lysine K) that has been reported to help avoid the immune response, which may compromise the effectiveness of current vaccines. A mutation in this same position is the E484Q (the Glutamic acid in position 484 has been changed by a Glutamine Q) that has been identified in the *delta* variant and produces a differently folded spike that seems to improve the binding to the host ACE2 receptor. The N501Y mutation (the Asparagine N in position 501 has been substituted by a Tyrosine Y) is present in the *alpha, beta* and *gamma* variants and is located in the receptor binding domain (RBD) of the spike protein that binds to the host ACE2 receptor. Thus, it has been reported to increase the binding affinity to this host receptor (Chand et al., 2020). The Serine at the 477 position, which is located in the RBD of the virus spike, seems to be a very flexible one and it has been found mutated to N (Asparagine) in the Spanish-variant, or to G (Glycine) in other variants. These mutations help to strengthen the binding to the ACE2 receptor in the host. Other mutations that have been detected in different variants are:

- the P681H (*alpha* variant) responsible for the exponential increase in cases in the UK and Ireland in late 2020 and then later worldwide in early 2021 as discussed in Chapter 4
- the L452R, P681R and the N440K mutations (*delta* variant) responsible for enhancing binding to the host ACE2 receptor that seems to be involved in the second surge of cases in India, also examined in Chapter 4.

---

news-medical.net/news/20210427/Triple-mutation-in-SARS-CoV-2-seen-in-second-wave-of-COVID-19-in-India.aspx

SARS-CoV-2 detection

Once the pandemic was clearly expanding, there was a need for fast and cheap techniques that would allow early detection to identify whether a person had been infected by the virus or not. The European Centre for Disease prevention and Control (ECDC) together with the WHO have recently published a report describing the plethora of methods available.[17] In this chapter we will only mention two of these methods, which are the most commonly used, RT-PCR and Rapid Antigen detection; additionally, detection by the analysis of waste waters will be briefly discussed.

Taking advantage of a known technique, the Polymerase Chain Reaction or PCR technique, it was possible to develop a quick and reliable method for the detection of SARS-CoV-2. This PCR technique consists of amplifying (i.e. making multiple copies) small sections of DNA to obtain a sufficient amount for their identification. This technique was discovered and established by Kary B. Mullis who won the Chemistry Nobel Prize in 1993 for this achievement.[18] The PCR procedure follows several cycles each comprising of two steps. First, denaturation of DNA takes place by heating the sample, this means that the two strands that form the double helix of DNA are separated by heat. Next, in the annealing and extension step, the system cools down and the enzyme called polymerase synthesizes two new DNA strands using as a template those strands that were separated in the denaturation step; in that way the original DNA is duplicated. The two steps can be repeated over and over (up to 30 or 40 times) producing more than 1 billion copies in just a few hours.[19] This technique can be applied to identify DNA of different microorganisms such as bacteria or viruses. In the case of SARS-CoV-2, since it is an RNA containing virus, a variant of PCR needs to be used: the so-called reverse transcriptase PCR (RT-PCR). This modified assay requires an enzyme (reverse transcriptase) to transform the RNA of the virus into DNA and then this viral DNA is amplified as per the normal PCR technique. RT-PCR tests are considered the 'gold standard' for clinical diagnostic detection of SARS-CoV-2. In practical terms, if the sample taken from the nares of the person being tested contains the virus, there would be viral RNA present; by using the RT-PCR, that RNA will be transformed into viral DNA, amplified and positively identified.

---

17 https://www.ecdc.europa.eu/en/publications-data/methods-detection-and-identification-sars-cov-2-variants

18 https://www.nobelprize.org/prizes/chemistry/1993/mullis/facts/

19 https://www.genome.gov/about-genomics/fact-sheets/Polymerase-Chain-Reaction-Fact-Sheet

A quicker, cheaper, but less accurate method of detection is the (Rapid) Antigen detection test. This test can identify the presence of the virus and help to decrease transmission through early detection. This methodology detects the presence or absence of 'antigens' (i.e. a protein from the virus) in the body, but not antibodies (they take longer to develop) or the viral nucleic acid (i.e. RNA in the case of SARS-CoV-2). The results of these immunochromatographic assays can be seen after 5 to 30 minutes and the test does not require specific training. Their sensitivity can vary because it depends on the levels of viral antigens which are different at the beginning, middle, and late parts of the infection; thus, false negatives can be obtained (Feng et al., 2020). These tests were already known as diagnostic tools for influenza and other infections of the respiratory system.

The third detection method is the analysis of waste waters in populated areas. Considering that many infected subjects are asymptomatic, the RT-PCR and antigen methods are not always useful, thus increasing the risk of transmission. To be able to identify all infected cases requires a large infrastructure that is not always accessible in economically depressed areas. However, analysing the sewage in particular areas of population is an easy way to identify the presence of the virus in that area and anticipating its spread (Eftekhari et al., 2021). The SARS-CoV-2 can be detected in the faeces and urine of infected patients and it has been reported that this virus survives for a long time in its active form. Therefore, identifying the presence of the virus in infected areas by analysing a community's wastewater can help to quickly determine areas of high incidence of the virus facilitating decision making to reduce viral spread, particularly in geographically contained clusters.

COVID-19, the disease

We have seen so far how the SARS-CoV-2 virus enters the human host cells, how it replicates within the host, and how it can mutate to produce new more aggressive variants to overcome the immune response of the human body. But, how does COVID-19 develop as a disease? How is it identified? Which are the symptoms, risks and consequences?

COVID-19 can present in many different clinical forms including asymptomatic individuals. Depending on factors such as age (children are rarely infected, while severe forms happen in people >65 years old) or preconditions such as diabetes, cardiovascular disease, chronic respiratory disease or cancer, COVID-19 can evolve from a mild condition to a very severe and lethal illness.[20] Once the virus enters the body there is an incubation period after which two possible scenarios can arise:

(i) an upper respiratory tract infection typically observed in young patients that results in positive outcomes or

(ii) a lower respiratory tract infection (pneumonia-like) usually seen in older patients or patients with underlying conditions that results in a very serious to fatal disease (Gautret et al., 2020).

In the early days of the pandemic, it was thought that the most common way of transmission for SARS-CoV-2 was through surfaces and hence an emphasis was made on hygiene (hands and surfaces) and distancing. Later on, it was confirmed that the main route of transmission is through respiratory droplets (i.e. aerosols) containing the virus, which can be inhaled or get in touch with the eyes, nose, or mouth of a person who is at a distance of less of 1.5 meters. Accordingly, the use of face masks and distancing were strongly encouraged.

Once the virus has entered the human, there is an incubation time between 2 and 14 days and then the symptoms start to appear. However, it needs to be emphasized that asymptomatic cases have often been seen: these patients will not suffer from the disease but still will be able to transmit it to other more vulnerable subjects. The WHO estimates that around 80 % of COVID-19 infections are mild or asymptomatic, whereas the CDC indicates that due to the lack of routine testing it is not possible to clearly establish the occurrence of asymptomatic infection. However, based on their data of PCR and serologic testing they estimate that the number of actual cases is larger than those reported.[21]

Typical symptoms observed in COVID-19 are fever, cough, difficulty breathing, loss of sense of smell (anosmia)[22] and/or taste (ageusia), among others. Fever is considered when the body temperature is over 38 °C and it is the typical response of the body to any type of infection (viral or bacterial). Cough and difficulty breathing are expected symptoms since the virus enters mostly through the upper respiratory system (nose and mouth) and has affinity for the ACE2 receptors in the lung cells where it replicates. However, the symptoms associated with loss of sense of smell and/or taste are unique to this disease and were unexpected. It has been estimated that anosmia and ageusia occur in around 53 % of COVID-19 patients and these two symptoms have been used to diagnose the

---

20 https://news.cornell.edu/stories/2020/04/why-covid-19-mild-some-deadly-others
21 https://www.cdc.gov/coronavirus/2019-ncov/hcp/clinical-guidance-management-patients.html
22 https://www.news-medical.net/health/COVID-19-and-Smell-Loss-(Anosmia).aspx

illness with a certainty of 67% over the PCR detected cases (Boudjema et al., 2020). Butowt et al. (2020) suggest that the global incidence of the D614G mutation is related to the frequency of anosmia and ageusia in COVID-19 patients, and they propose that the higher binding of the RBD of the spike protein to the ACE2 receptor of the host results in a higher infection of the olfactory epithelium. All these symptoms contribute to the diagnosis and may be mild with no treatment required except for some antiviral therapy that could reduce the time for recovery and progression to the most severe disease. Patients that can keep the viral infection to this level have a very good prognosis and are likely to recover without needing hospitalization.

However, in some patients the infection evolves to a second stage affecting the lungs producing inflammation (i. e. pulmonary disease). This results in pneumonia and hypoxia (i. e. lack of oxygen) and requires hospitalization. Potential therapies at this stage are, for example, the broad-spectrum antibiotic rifampicin, the newly developed antiviral remdesivir and broadly acting anti-inflammatory agents such as dexamethasone, which has proved to be very efficient in controlling the disease at this stage. However, if the hypoxia cannot be controlled with these therapies, mechanical ventilation (i. e. ventilators) could be required.

If the infection has not been controlled at this second stage, the disease will move to a more severe stage characterized by extrapulmonary systemic hyperinflammation that probably will require the patient to be moved to an intensive care unit (ICU). A minority of patients reach this stage and they will suffer a noticeable decrease in T-cells, which are those in charge of 'defending' the human body from the 'attack' of different microorganisms. Additionally, an increase in different inflammation related proteins such as cytokines (i. e. IL-2, IL-6 or IL-7), macrophage inflammatory protein or ferritin is observed. This is known as the 'cytokine storm' and results from a strong immune response towards the own body (autoimmune response), killing not only the virus but also cells and tissues driving to organ failure, sepsis and death. Cytokine responses were already known in autoimmune diseases such as lupus or arthritis and they also can take place in certain cancer therapies and influenza infections. Most patients suffering COVID-19 recover completely from the disease, but patients with underlying conditions should be more closely monitored since they can more easily move to the second and third stages of the disease, which are those with poorer prognoses.

An additional problem that has been identified worldwide is the post-COVID conditions (known as Long COVID) that have been identified in some patients. These comprise several health problems and last for more than four weeks after being infected by the virus and have been classified as Long COVID, Multiorgan effects or Effects resulting from COVID-19 treatment or hospitalization.[23] Long COVID can occur in patients who showed serious, mild or lack of symptoms and presents a variety of symptoms such as fatigue, loss of smell/taste, dizziness, difficulty concentrating, headaches, depression/anxiety or muscle pain. Those patients suffering multiorgan effects post-COVID can present conditions affecting different organ functions, by inflammation or autoimmune responses. Finally, the longer-term effects of the antiviral or anti-inflammatory treatments given to COVID-19 patients as well as the effects of long hospitalization or ICU care and post-traumatic stress disorder (PTSD) can be included within the Long COVID conditions.

From a scientific vantage, treating a viral infection is a fascinating challenge with huge rewards if a solution is found. In the remainder of the chapter, we discuss the steps to put a drug on the market from drug design to marketing. Thereafter, we examine antiviral therapies to treat COVID-19 as well as vaccines to prevent it. For clarity, the reader should note that when we refer to antiviral drugs/therapies we are talking about treatments to stop the viral infection whereas vaccines are biological products that defend the body from the infection.

Treating COVID-19 infections: drug development

Knowledge of the replication cycle of a virus helps to identify potential 'targets' to develop antiviral drugs. Knowing proteins or enzymes required for the production of new virions opens up the possibility to develop small-molecules (drugs) that will interfere with those systems, thus stopping the reproduction of the virus, i.e. the infection. For example, the antiviral drug acyclovir, which is used to treat herpes simplex virus infections, blocks a specific enzyme of the virus (i.e. DNA polymerase). Even knowing the 'target' of a drug, the process required for the development of new therapeutic agents is very complex, time consuming and very expensive. Therefore, in the discovery of a drug or therapeutic agent we can consider two stages: that of 'design and synthesis' and that of 'development'. The first stage of 'design and synthesis' consists of three steps:
(i)   selection of the objective or 'target',
(ii) identification of a prototype or 'lead' compound that shows the biological activity we are looking for but is not yet suitable as a drug, and finally
(iii) optimisation of this 'lead' compound improving its efficacy and decreasing its toxicity.

---

23 https://www.cdc.gov/coronavirus/2019-ncov/long-term-effects.html

In the 'development' stage (Figure 2.8) we can distinguish between the:
(i)   pre-clinical studies,
(ii) the clinical trials and
(iii) the post-marketing vigilance.

Pre-clinical studies consist of *in vitro* assays (in 'naked' receptors, cells, or isolated tissues), followed by *in vivo* or animal tests (in rodents such as mice and rats, or rabbits). Four to six years of pre-clinical testing are usually required to identify acute and subacute animal toxicities and to establish the probable limits of the clinical dosage range by identifying the Maximum Tolerated Dose (MTD). Before starting the clinical trials, when the drug is going to be tested for the first time in humans, an Investigational New Drug (IND) application needs to be submitted to the corresponding regulatory agency (FDA or EMA) and only when this is approved, can Phase I begin.

Thus, in Phase 1 clinical trials the effects of the drug using different doses are determined in a small cohort of healthy volunteers (20 – 100). The most important aim of Phase I trials is to identify significant differences in the response to the drug's MTD between humans and animals. These trials are non-blind, which means that both the investigators and the subjects know what drug is taken (i.e. placebo, experimental or established drug). Different aspects of the absorption of the drug, its elimination from the body, half-life or metabolic transformations in the body are determined. Additionally, many predictable toxicities are detected, and different doses are explored in this phase; these studies are usually performed in research centres by clinical pharmacologists.

In Phase II clinical trials, the new drug is tested for the first time in patients suffering from the disease that is studied, and the objective is not only to determine safety, but also efficacy (Figure 2.8). Between 100 and 500 patients are considered for the study. A single-blind design is usually followed, utilizing an inert placebo and an already known drug (positive control) for the disease in addition to the agent under investigation. These trials are performed in special clinical centres and a wider range of toxicities may be detected.

Finally, during the Phase III clinical trials the drug is tested in a broader cohort of patients that could reach up to the thousands (Figure 2.8). Considering the information previously obtained in Phases I and II, these clinical trials need to be carefully designed in order to minimize the potential errors due to the 'placebo effect' or to the variable progression of the disease, among other factors. Therefore, double blind protocols are followed, which means that neither the evaluator nor the subject knows which item is being supplied and all the information is kept in a closed envelope during the whole trial. Considering the large number of patients involved in Phase III studies and the amount of data generated that must be analyzed, these trials are difficult to design, execute and finance. In general, the researchers behind these Phase III trials are specialists in the disease studied. At this point a New Drug Application must be submitted to the corresponding regulatory agency (i.e. FDA or EMA) with all the results obtained in the three phases of the clinical trials in order for the drug to be allowed into the general population.

Once 'approval to market' of a drug is obtained, and as soon as the drug is being prescribed for its use to the general population, Phase IV begins (Figure 2.8). This post marketing phase involves the final release of the new drug for general prescription, supervising that it is safe when used by many patients, and keeping track of any adverse reaction reported by health professionals (i.e. pharmacists and doctors). In this Phase IV surveillance, many important effects induced by the new drug, which were not detected in Phases I, II or III and have an incidence of 1:10,000 or less, are identified. The intellectual property of a new drug is usually protected by a patent even at the preclinical phase, the lifetime of a patent is 17–20 years and after that time any company may produce and market the drug. In other words, the period between the design of an active substance and when it reaches the public domain is usually very long and 20 years can easily pass by.

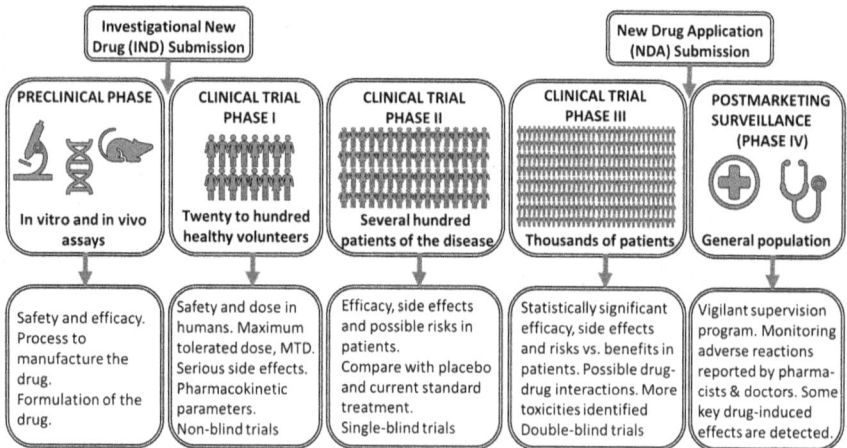

Investigational New Drug (IND) Submission			New Drug Application (NDA) Submission	
PRECLINICAL PHASE	CLINICAL TRIAL PHASE I	CLINICAL TRIAL PHASE II	CLINICAL TRIAL PHASE III	POSTMARKETING SURVEILLANCE (PHASE IV)
In vitro and in vivo assays	Twenty to hundred healthy volunteers	Several hundred patients of the disease	Thousands of patients	General population
Safety and efficacy. Process to manufacture the drug. Formulation of the drug.	Safety and dose in humans. Maximum tolerated dose, MTD. Serious side effects. Pharmacokinetic parameters. Non-blind trials	Efficacy, side effects and possible risks in patients. Compare with placebo and current standard treatment. Single-blind trials	Statistically significant efficacy, side effects and risks vs. benefits in patients. Possible drug-drug interactions. More toxicities identified Double-blind trials	Vigilant supervision program. Monitoring adverse reactions reported by pharmacists & doctors. Some key drug-induced effects are detected.

Figure 2.8: Development stage of a new drug indicating all the steps: preclinical studies, clinical trials (phase I, II and III) as well as the post-marketing vigilance phase IV. The points when an Investigational New Drug (NDI) application and a New Drug Application (NDA) are submitted are also indicated.

Treating COVID-19 infections: antiviral drugs

To date, no antiviral agent has exhibited full efficacy against SARS-CoV-2. Despite the fact that different vaccines are available, as discussed later, part of the population that suffers different immuno-compromised conditions will not be able to be vaccinated. To be immuno-compromised means that the immune system is not working properly; this can happen when the person either suffers from a disease, or receives a treatment that suppresses the immune system, such as patients with blood cancers, HIV or autoimmune conditions, or well recipients of an organ transplant taking immunosuppressant drugs. As stated by Dr Fauci 'It is clear that if you are on immunosuppressant agents, history tells us that you are not going to have as robust a response as if you had an intact immune system that was not being compromised.'[24] Therefore, there is an urgent need to find efficient drugs to treat COVID-19, which continues to be a worldwide threat.

Even though only one drug has been approved to date to treat some of the stages of COVID-19 (i.e. remdesivir), existing drugs already approved by the FDA/EMA for other illnesses are being surveyed as potential treatments for the disease. These therapeutic agents are known as 'repurposing' drugs, and several are being studied as potential treatments for COVID-19. Considering the replication cycle of the SARS-CoV-2 virus shown in Figure 2.7, there are several small molecules (novel and repurposing drugs) being explored as potential anti-COVID-19 therapies; next we will briefly discuss some of these research initiatives. Two known drugs, *camostat* and *nafamostat*, have been proposed to interfere with the viral-host fusion, stopping the entry of the virus into the host cell by inhibiting the TMPRSS2 protease involved in this process. Camostat is commercialized by Ono Pharmaceuticals in Japan for the treatment of chronic pancreatitis and reflux esophagitis, whereas nafamostat has also been used for the treatment of pancreatitis and is known to be a short-acting anticoagulant. Because camostat and nafamostat have shown very potent anti-SARS-CoV-2 activity *in vitro* and *in vivo* in mice (Hoffman et al., 2020b), both drugs have been included in several clinical trials.[25] The results reported so far for camostat show that it is not very effective in hospitalized patients, but the authors do not exclude the possibility that administration of high dose TMPRSS2 inhibitors such as camostat or nafamostat could have a positive effect in the early stages of COVID-19 (Gunst, 2021), decreasing the risk of the most severe stage of the disease as de-

---

24 https://www.ajmc.com/view/ash-2020-covid-19-and-hematology
25 https://public.tableau.com/app/profile/marinamarin/viz/covidTrials/COVID-19Clinical TrialsExplorer

fined before in this chapter. The advantage of these drugs is that they block the host enzyme that activates the viral spike (i. e. TMPRSS2) and, therefore, they are equally active versus any SARS-CoV-2 variant.

As shown in Figure 2.7, once the virus has entered the host cell, viral genome activation takes place in the cytoplasm by the action of different enzymes. Viral RNA-dependent RNA polymerases manage transcription and replication of the viral genome; hence, blocking the action of these enzymes stops the replication cycle of the virus. An example of this type of drug is *remdesivir* (brand name Ve-klury), an adenosine nucleoside ProTide prodrug (technologically pioneered by Prof. Chris McGuigan, see Mehellou et al., 2017), that was originally developed by the company Gilead to treat Ebola virus (Figure 2.9). This compound under-goes a series of chemical changes in the body to produce the actual drug that looks like a nucleoside triphosphate (RNA building blocks), which is the actual inhibitor of the RNA polymerase. In April 2020, the company Gilead started Phase III clinical trials to investigate the toxicity and efficacy of remdesivir in COVID-19 patients with moderate to severe illness. By May of that year, the EMA started to review the use of this drug for the treatment of COVID-19 and rec-ommends its compassionate use in patients who are not on mechanical ventila-tion. Between May and June several countries had approved its use and by the end of May the first generic version of remdesivir was sold in Bangladesh. The FDA granted full approval to remdesivir by the end of October 2020, making it the first treatment for COVID-19 that has been approved.

Another polymerase inhibitor that has been explored as an antiviral for SARS-CoV-2 is *favipiravir* (brand name Avigan), a known antiviral treatment for influenza (Shiraki and Daikoku, 2020) produced by Japan's Fujifilm (through its subsidiary Toyama Chemical) (Figure 2.9). This compound is also a prodrug that is transformed into a nucleoside triphosphate in the body, which inhibits RNA-dependent RNA polymerase enzymatic activity. Favipiravir was approved for influenza treatment in Japan in 2014 and it became a generic drug by 2019. By mid-March 2020, trials with this drug were performed in a small group of pa-tients in Wuhan and Shenzhen and found that it reduced pneumonia symptoms. In early May 2020, the pharma company Glenmark in India received approval and started Phase III clinical trials with favipiravir. In June 2020, the Ministry of Health in Russia approved favipiravir as a COVID-19 therapy. After several clin-ical trials in India, favipiravir was approved for the treatment of mild to moder-ate COVID-19 in this country by August 2020; at the same time the US FDA ex-panded the Phase II trials performed by Appili Therapeutics to use favipiravir in COVID-19 prevention at long-term care facilities.

After the genome activation, translation of the viral RNA produces large pro-teins that need to be 'cut' into the corresponding enzymes and structural pro-

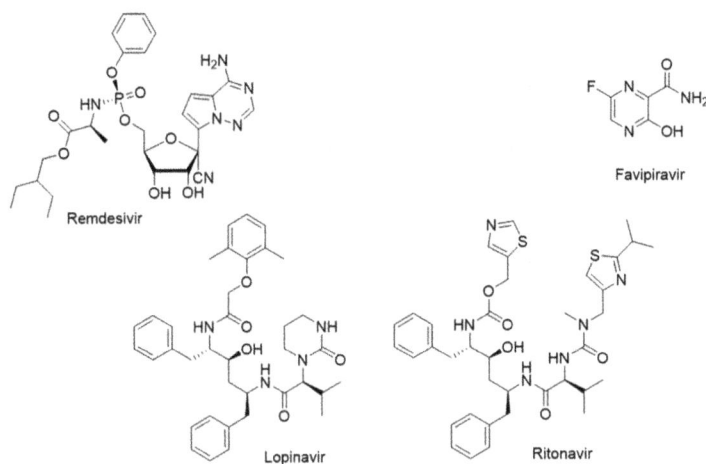

Figure 2.9: Structures of some of the drugs approved or experimentally studied as COVID-19 treatments.

teins for the new viruses (Figure 2.7). This process is performed by proteases and, in the case of the SARS-CoV-2 virus, the main protease (M^{pro}) has been chosen a target for antiviral therapies. A combination of two known protease inhibitors used to treat HIV infections and developed by AbbVie was tested for their potential as COVID-19 therapies, *lopinavir* and *ritonavir* (Kaletra) (Figure 2.9). However, while a study by Cao et al. (2020) suggested that the use of Kaletra in seriously ill COVID-19 patients did not shorten the hospitalisation time or lower mortality rates, a clinical trial performed by Lancaster University considered this treatment successful. Combining of lopinavir with other therapies (hydroxychloroquine, interferon or ribavirin) was also explored, indicating some positive results in patients with mild to moderate cases. Finally, in July 2020, WHO advised discontinuation of the lopinavir/ritonavir combination as therapy for COVID-19. Other M^{pro} inhibitors such as danoprevir, boceprevir or ebselen have been explored as potential treatments for COVID-19 with mixed results.

Further, drugs with either proven antiviral response (i. e. elsulfavirine or brequinar), known effect on lung conditions (i. e. ANG-3777 or ifenprodil), or vascular stability activity (i. e. razuprotafib) have been tested to treat COVID-19. Nonetheless, no final positive results have been reported at the time of writing. Additionally, considering that one of the critical points in COVID-19 is the 'cytokine storm' that produces a strong inflammatory response, different anti-inflammatory drugs have been explored as COVID-19 therapies. Some examples are:

- *auxora*, an inhibitor of calcium-release activated calcium-channel, which has been tested in COVID-19 patients with severe pneumonia or acute respiratory distress syndrome (ARDS);
- *thymosin beta 4*, a therapeutic peptide with potential use in multiple sclerosis because of its regenerative properties, which is a strong anti-inflammatory agent;
- the sphingosine kinase-2 (SK2) selective inhibitor *opaganib*, which is an investigational drug for inflammatory indications;
- *ensifentrine*, a novel inhibitor of both phosphodiesterase 3 and 4 with bronchodilator and anti-inflammatory properties;
- the cysteine derivative *bucillamine*, which may have anti-inflammatory activity through an unknown mechanism of action;
- the antagonist of known inflammatory agents such as neurokinin 1 and substance-P *tradipitant*;
- the palmitoyl-glycerol derivative *EC-18* that is being studied to prevent ARDS due to COVID-19 pneumonia; or
- a marine product, *plitidepsin*, showing very good activity against SARS-CoV-2 infections by interacting with the host protein eEF1 A (eukaryotic translation elongation factor 1 A) (White et al., 2021).

Treating COVID-19 infections: biologic therapies

Considering the advances in knowledge of the human immune system during the last 20 years and that behind many diseases there is an immune pathogenesis, new types of treatment have been developed: biologic therapies. Examples of these treatments are monoclonal antibodies and fusion proteins and they incorporate recognition components that function as antibodies. According to the NIH/NCI, biological therapies or *biologics* use compounds produced by living organisms to treat diseases.[26] These biologics can be natural or prepared in the laboratory and they differ from the 'small-molecule' drugs in their size (biologics are larger than small-molecule drugs) as well as in their nature (biologics are extracted or based on compounds existing in living organisms, while small-molecule drugs are chemically derived).

We have talked about the immune system several times in this chapter, but what does this immune system entail? There are two types of immunity in the body, innate and lymphocyte-driven or adaptive:

---

26 https://www.cancer.gov/publications/dictionaries/cancer-terms/def/biological-therapy

- *Innate immunity* acts immediately after the body has been in contact with the pathogens (e.g. viruses, bacteria, parasites or any foreign particles) and it is nonspecific, meaning it is the same for a virus as for a foreign particle for example. It consists of physical barriers (e.g. skin, saliva, or inflammation) and types of white blood cells, or leukocytes such as phagocytic cells, macrophages, mast cells or neutrophils, among others.
- *Adaptive immunity* is slower, is triggered by the recognition of an antigen and depends on a number of cells: B- and T-cells. B-cells are formed and matured in the bone-marrow and recognize antigens. T-cells are formed in the bone-marrow but matured in the thymus, where they develop receptors (i.e. T-cell receptors, CD4, CD8), and they recognize antigens that are bound to certain receptor molecules.

The fight against COVID-19 has mobilized research in the field of biologics towards SARS-CoV-2 antiviral therapies. Almost all ongoing novel biologic therapeutic efforts are directed to use antibodies that recognize the RBD of the virus' spike or to try to prevent the infection. Similar to remdesivir being the only drug approved by the FDA as a COVID-19 therapy, there are two biologic combinations that have been also approved by the FDA, *casirivimab + imdevimab* (REGN-COV2) and *bamlanivimab + etesevimab*.

Since March 2020, many biological therapies, which were already known as treatments for other conditions, have been explored as antivirals for COVID-19. For example:
- the companies Sanofi and Regeneron Pharmaceutical explored the potential of the monoclonal antibody *sarilumab* (inhibitor of the interleukin 6 receptor, IL-6), which is a treatment for rheumatoid arthritis, in the care of severe COVID-19 patients.
- Roche investigated *tocilizumab* (a treatment for rheumatoid arthritis) in COVID-19 patients with pneumonia,
- Altasciences as well as Roivant studied *gimsilumab* to treat the ARDS in COVID-19,
- InflaRx explored *vilobelimab* (IFX-1) for severe COVID-19,
- Novant Health with CytoDyn tested *leronlimab* (a known treatment for breast cancer),
- Humanigen studied *lenzilumab* in COVID-19 patients, and
- R-Pharm with Cromos Pharma performed trials with *olokizumab* and RPH-104 in patients with severe COVID-19.

The company Eli Lilly investigated their experimental monoclonal antibodies LY-CoV555 (*bamlanivimab*) and LY-CoV016 (*etesevimab*), which in combination gave excellent results in reducing hospitalizations and deaths in high-risk COVID-19 patients. Based on these results the FDA and the EMA granted emergency use authorization. Meanwhile, Regeneron explored a dual antibody cocktail with *casirivimab* plus *imdevimab* with very successful outcomes; this combination, commercialized as REGN-COV2, got a lot of publicity since it was disclosed to be the therapy given to US President Donald Trump and was approved for emergency use by the FDA in November 2020.[27]

A word on COVID-19 clinical trials

At the end of 2020, there were 3,418 on-going COVID-19 trials with different therapies,[28] and some examples will be discussed next. At the beginning of the pandemic (March 2020), the WHO started a clinical trial ('Solidarity') which by October had more than 11,000 participants in 30 countries testing the efficacy of drugs known to attack certain viral targets such as viral polymerases (*remdesivir*) or HIV proteases (*lopinavir* and *ritonavir*), busting the immune system (*interferon*) or anti-malarial agents thought to have an anti-inflammatory effect (*hydroxychloroquine*). Unfortunately, it was found that none of these drugs had a real effect in improving the outcome of hospital patients with COVID-19.

In May 2020, an observational study carried out by Hackensack Meridian Heath showed lack of efficacy of *hydroxychloroquine* among COVID-19 patients in hospitals but indicated that the biological *tocilizumab* improved survival. Similarly, as part of the RECOVERY clinical trial, Oxford University found in June 2020 that *hydroxychloroquine* had no clinical benefit in hospitalized patients.

As stated before, an explosive immune response of the body (i.e. 'cytokine storm') can be one of the problems found in COVID-19 since it affects healthy tissues as well as infected cells. For that reason, in the mentioned RECOVERY trial it was found that immuno-suppressive agents such as the broad-spectrum anti-inflammatory *dexamethasone* reduced deaths in patients needing ventilators or supplemental oxygen. Another internationally driven trial ('Remap-Cap'), aimed to test the efficacy of biologics such as *tocilizumab* and *sarilumab* that block the immune protein interleukin-6 (IL-6), found that these treatments reduced deaths in COVID-19 critical patients.

---

27 https://www.cnbc.com/2020/11/21/covid-treatment-fda-authorizes-regeneron-drug-used-by-trump.html
28 https://public.tableau.com/app/profile/marinamarin/viz/covidTrials/COVID-19ClinicalTrialsExplorer

Preventing COVID-19 infections: vaccines

Since almost the beginning of the pandemic, many pharmaceutical companies and research groups around the world raced to find a vaccine to protect and prevent people from getting the SARS-CoV-2 virus; it is now widely accepted that the only way to free the world from the COVID-19 pandemic is by means of extensive immunization against the virus using effective vaccines. But what is a vaccine? According to the CDC, a vaccine is a biological 'product that stimulates a person's immune system to produce immunity to a specific disease, protecting the person from that disease'.[29] Vaccines are given to train our immune system to fight against pathogens in future infections.

Vaccination is the most effective way to protect the population against dangerous viral and bacterial diseases before getting infected. Once a person is exposed to a pathogen, the body responds by activating the immune system by generating T-cells and/or neutralizing antibodies to counterattack the pathogen. A vaccine stimulates the normal human response against infection (e.g. T-cells and/or neutralizing antibodies) to build resistance to specific pathogens, making the body's immune system stronger.

In the previous section we have seen how there are different steps in the development of drugs and how there are three clinical trial phases when a drug is tested in humans (Phases I to III). Similar to these three clinical phases to establish drugs' safety and efficacy in humans, there are three clinical trials phases in the development of vaccines (Figure 2.10). Thus, during Phase 1, small groups of volunteers receive the trial vaccine. In Phase 2, the study is extended, and the vaccine is administered to people with specific characteristics (e.g. age, physical health) common to those for whom the new vaccine is aimed. Finally, in Phase 3, the vaccine is given to a large cohort of people (i.e. thousands) and tested for efficacy and safety (Figure 2.10). Like the development process already described for drugs, vaccines undergo Phase 4 monitoring controls after the vaccine has been approved and licensed. This is the reason why the secondary effects of the AstraZeneca and Johnson & Johnson vaccines (blood clot forming) were identified while the vaccine was already being administered to the general population.

The effort in developing a vaccine for the COVID-19 pandemic is unprecedented in terms of both scale and speed. However, these fast discovery and production processes have cast doubt about the 'quality' or safety of the vaccines produced. These doubts are completely unfounded since the discovery process

---

29 https://www.cdc.gov/vaccines/vac-gen/imz-basics.htm

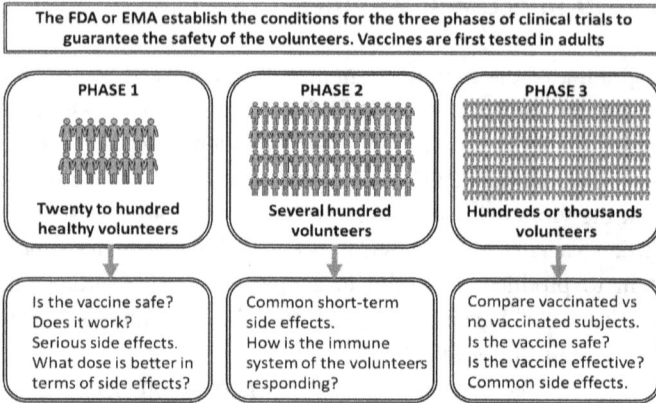

The FDA or EMA establish the conditions for the three phases of clinical trials to guarantee the safety of the volunteers. Vaccines are first tested in adults

PHASE 1	PHASE 2	PHASE 3
Twenty to hundred healthy volunteers	Several hundred volunteers	Hundreds or thousands volunteers
Is the vaccine safe? Does it work? Serious side effects. What dose is better in terms of side effects?	Common short-term side effects. How is the immune system of the volunteers responding?	Compare vaccinated vs no vaccinated subjects. Is the vaccine safe? Is the vaccine effective? Common side effects.

Figure 2.10: Different phases in the development of a new vaccine before it is licensed and reaches the general public.

and clinical trials in humans have followed all the controls established by the regulatory bodies and the speed of the process can be explained by a much larger amount of funds dedicated to this as will be discussed in following chapters. Similarly, the production and control of the vaccines licensed have followed the same controls as any previous vaccine, that is, the vaccines are prepared in lots, every lot is tested in terms of safety, quality and potency, and the factories where these lots are prepared are inspected often by regulatory bodies such as FDA or EMA (Figure 2.11).

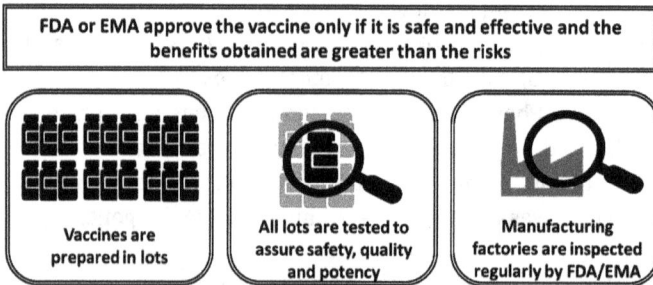

FDA or EMA approve the vaccine only if it is safe and effective and the benefits obtained are greater than the risks

Vaccines are prepared in lots	All lots are tested to assure safety, quality and potency	Manufacturing factories are inspected regularly by FDA/EMA

Figure 2.11: Vaccine production control after being licensed.

We have already described how the spike protein of the virus is a fundamental viral element for SARS-CoV-2 to be able to enter (i.e. infect) a host cell. This spike protein has been identified as the most important antigen of the virus and it has been found that antibodies recognize a specific part of this spike (i.e. RBD) that is responsible for binding to the host receptor (i.e. ACE2) (Figure 2.12-A). This demonstrates that this antigen, the viral spike protein, is the best target for a vaccine and, based on this, different approaches to a vaccine for COVID-19 have been pursued. Hence, we can distinguish different types of vaccine such as (i) inactivated virus, (ii) viral vector, (iii) mRNA and (iv) viral protein subunits vaccines (Figure 2.12-B).

First, the *inactivated virus* vaccines consist of viruses that have been chemically inactivated or are dead but that can still induce the production of the antigen (i.e. the spike in the case of SARS-CoV-2) (Figure 2.12-Bi). When administered, the human cells use the genetic material of those inactivated/dead viruses to

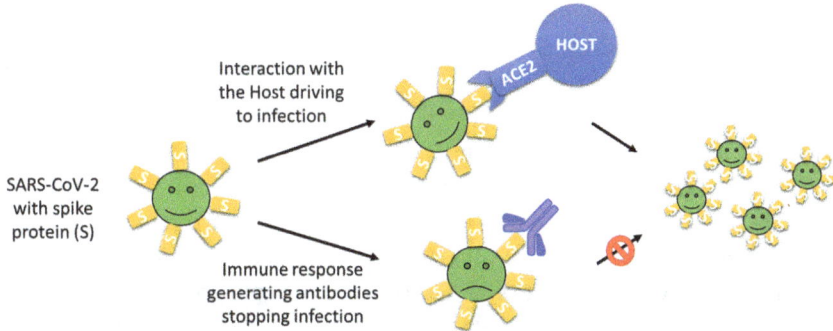

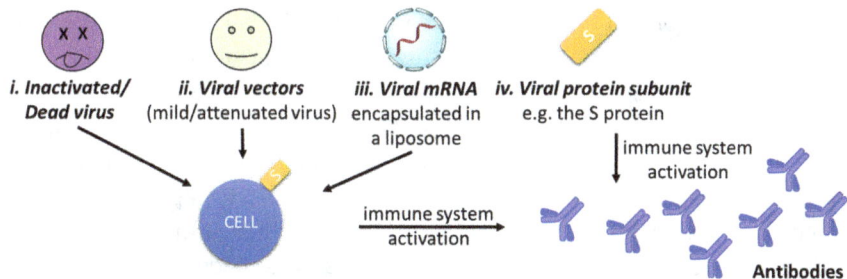

Figure 2.12: A: SARS-CoV-2 has a protein spike (S) in its surface that helps the virus to interact and infect the host human cells; alternatively, this S protein can trigger the immune response in the body. **B:** Different vaccines make use of (i) *inactivated virus*, (ii) *viral vectors*, or (iii) *viral mRNA* to make human cells to produce the S protein thus activating the immune system, other vaccines (iv) use *viral protein(s)* to activate the immune system; activation of the immune system produces antibodies to defend the body from future viral infections.

produce the spike protein, thus triggering the immune response. Two Chinese companies, Sinopharm and Sinovac, and one Indian company, Bharat Biotech, have developed their vaccines following this approach. Both Chinese companies have used different inactivated strains of the SARS-CoV-2 (HB02 and CN02, respectively) prepared from Vero cells, which are epithelial cells isolated from the African green monkey kidney and used in general to prepare vaccines. Both vaccines, named BBIBP-CorV and CoronaVac, respectively, were approved by the WHO for their use in May and June 2021. Regarding the vaccine developed by Bharat Biotech (Covaxin), it is prepared with killed coronaviruses isolated by India's National Institute of Virology; these dead viruses are still recognized by the immune cells triggering the production of antibodies against the virus. Covaxin phase 3 trials' results so far are showing an 81% efficacy and in January 2021 India's regulators gave it an emergency approval status even before this phase 3 has been completed. There are experts who consider this highly dangerous because the vaccine is not completely studied; however, manufacturers and regulators manifest that Covaxin is safe and provides good protection against SARS-CoV-2.

Second, the most common approach to the SARS-CoV-2 vaccines developed so far is the use of a *viral vector* (Figure 2.12-Bii). The idea behind this type of vaccine is to manipulate a mild or attenuated virus (for example adenoviruses, which are the viruses that produce the common cold) to express the antigen of interest, in this case the spike protein as already mentioned. When administered, these mild viruses infect cells that produce the spike proteins, which are then recognized by the immune cells producing the corresponding immune response. The three companies that have used this methodology to develop a vaccine for COVID-19 are AstraZeneca/Oxford (ChAdOx1 or Covidshield), Jansen/Johnson & Johnson (Ad26.CoV2.S) and the Moscow's Gamaleya Institute (Sputnik V). While Covidshield contains adenoviruses from chimpanzees as viral vectors, Ad26.CoV2.S uses a harmless human adenovirus (Ad26) and Sputnik V uses two human adenoviruses as vectors (Ad5 and Ad26). Despite showing very good efficacy, controversy has followed these three vaccines. In the case of the AstraZeneca and Johnson & Johnson vaccines, the issue has been the appearance of rare blood clots in a small number of vaccinated people. Different theories have been proposed to explain this secondary effect such as the antibody response against the platelet activating factor PF4 which coordinates blood clotting (Greinacher et al., 2021), or the fact that the adenoviruses used as the vector replicate in the nucleus instead of the cytoplasm of the host cell, thus producing soluble spike proteins that can drive to blood clots (Kowarz et al., 2021). The debate around the Sputnik V vaccine is more related to its development; thus, the administration of this vaccine to the public in Russia started without a detailed animal study with primates and before the clinical trials were finalized. All data from pre-clinical or phase 1/2 trials have not yet been fully disclosed, but the results so far seen from phase 3 are very promising (Baraniuk, 2021). All of these vaccines require two doses except for that of Johnson & Johnson.

Third, the most novel method in SARS-CoV-2 immunization is that of the *mRNA vaccines*, which have been developed and commercialized by Pfizer/BioNTech (named BNT162b2), Moderna (mRNA-1273) and CureVac (CVnCoV) (Creech et al., 2021) (Figure 2.12-Biii). These vaccines contain messenger RNA (mRNA) inside a lipid nanoparticle that drives the nucleic acid to the host cell cytoplasm where is translated into the spike protein, which will move to the surface of the cell where it triggers the immune response. Only the vaccines from Pfizer and Moderna have been commercialized, they require two doses, and show a very good efficacy from the first dose and few secondary effects. Their only problem is the need for very low temperatures for their conservation. The vaccine from CureVac has recently lost the race since after phase 3 clinical trials it showed only a 47 % efficacy.[30]

Fourth, the use of a *viral protein subunit* to develop a vaccine takes advantage of the actual spike protein that can be prepared using some cell-based systems and when given to humans is recognized by the immune system starting a response to generate antibodies (Figure 2.12-Biv). An example of this type of vaccine is NVX-CoV2373 developed by Novavax, which uses recombinant full-length spike protein in a nanoparticle. This vaccine seems to have a good efficacy after two doses. Even though all clinical phases are already completed, the company is still waiting for approval.

As mentioned, many vaccines are being developed and some of them, which are in different stages of clinical trials, include:
- a vaccine developed by Hyderabad-based Biological E in collaboration with Dynavax and Baylor College of Medicine,
- mRNA vaccines from Bayern, Sanofi or Genova in collaboration with HDT Biotech Corporation (HGCO19),
- nasal vaccines by Bharat BioTech or by Intravacc,
- second-generation COVID-19 vaccines developed by CureVac with GlaxoSmithKline based on new mRNA backbones aiming for potential protection against multiple infectious diseases,
- Sinopharm's and Kangtai Biological's vaccines developed in China, or

---

30 https://www.curevac.com/en/2021/06/16/curevac-provides-update-on-phase-2b-3-trial-of-first-generation-covid-19-vaccine-candidate-cvncov/

- those developed in the Centro Nacional de Biotecnología in Spain (CNB-CSIC) such as the vaccine developed by the Spanish virologist Ramon Enjuanes, which uses their own methodology of 'synthetic virions' that contain attenuated viral RNA, and the one developed by Mariano Esteban, which is based in a very weakened vector virus (i. e. vaccinia virus) with DNA encoding the spike protein.[31]

Distribution and administration of the vaccines have been the object of many complications since vaccines started to be approved for the prevention of COVID-19. In terms of production/distribution, by December 2020 the US had bought 200 million doses of the Pfizer vaccine,[32] monopolizing production. Additionally, issues of production and distribution of the AstraZeneca vaccine brought the EU to take legal action against the company 'for not respecting its vaccine supply contract and for not having a "reliable" plan to ensure timely deliveries' as examined in more detail in Chapters 3 and 4.[33] Regarding the administration, the appearance of the mentioned rare secondary effects with the AstraZeneca and Johnson & Johnson vaccines, led to a halt in their use for the vaccination of the population under 40 – 60 years old (depending on the country). Additionally, in the particular case of AstraZeneca, which requires two doses, a disjunctive arose regarding what vaccine to use as the second dose in those people who had taken AstraZeneca as a first dose and were under the age limit established for safe use. On the one hand, the WHO and EMA recommended continuing with the same vaccine following protocol; however, countries such as Germany and France unilaterally decided to change the second dose to an mRNA based vaccine (i. e. Pfizer or Moderna), and countries such as Spain or Canada gave the population aged under 60 the option to choose AstraZeneca for the second dose or an mRNA vaccine. This decision may be based not only in the potential secondary effects mentioned, but also in the possibility of shortages of the AstraZeneca vaccine due to production issues.[34] Even though there is no evidence that mixing vaccine types for the first and second doses may be dangerous, there has not been a proper clinical trial carried out at the time of writing to support this approach: only studies in small groups have been performed which are not statistically significant.

31 https://www.csic.es/en/palabras-clave/vacuna-espanola
32 https://www.pfizer.com/news/press-release/press-release-detail/pfizer-and-biontech-supply-us-100-million-additional-doses
33 https://www.bbc.com/news/56483766
34 https://www.nytimes.com/2021/06/02/world/americas/canada-vaccine-mixing.html

Conclusions

In this chapter we have presented a brief introduction about the present COVID-19 pandemic not being the first one (or the last), the structure and replication of viruses (with a particular emphasis on SARS-CoV-2), and how COVID-19 develops as a disease. Additionally, we have presented how to develop antiviral treatments (small molecule drugs or biologic therapies) and which ones are being explored as treatments for COVID-19. Finally, a discussion about the different types of vaccines and their development has been included.

In the wake of this discussion, in the next chapter we will underline the significance of public policy responses in the absence of antivirals and/or vaccination. Two arguments will be made. First, we will argue that policy matters: while history has shown that countries alone cannot predict novel viruses from emerging per se, public policy choices made to control, contain, treat and prevent their spread are crucial, as seen recently in both SARS and the Swine Flu pandemics (Crawford, 2018, 128). Thus, public policy is important because it allows for 'control' of viruses before antiviral drugs and vaccines can be developed. Second, despite the significance of policy choices made by states, COVID-19 demonstrates that governments worldwide lack knowledge of what to do in a pandemic and the need for a theoretical conceptualization to guide states. Every pandemic has cultural, economic political, social and demographic effects (McMillen, 2016, 11). This begs for a strategy to not only spot an emerging infection, but also *deal* with emerging infections: this requires a government policy blueprint of what to do and what not to do, coupled with analysis of what has gone right, what could go better, and how should 'scientific criteria' inform 'political' decisions.

Chapter 3
Conceptualizing the four phases of a state's public policy responses during a pandemic: anticipating, containing, controlling and opening-up

Introduction

Covid-19 has caused an unprecedented health and economic crisis that governments faced without having a roadmap to tell them 'what policies to do' during a pandemic. This chapter develops that roadmap. This theoretical conceptualization of what governments should do when faced with any pandemic can be used by any reader to better understand developments in any state, anytime, during any pandemic. The typology thus serves as a blueprint for countries developing public policies when there is no immediate rapid scientific solution with a vaccine or antiviral. It also considers key points when countries rollout any antiviral or vaccine treatments when opening up society. As the experience of COVID-19 demonstrated, public policies are important: the recent pandemic acutely showed that '... when the going gets tough, the public relies on governments, not markets, to come to the rescue' (Mazey and Richardson, 2020, 568).

There are two main parts to this chapter. In the first, we take a historical look at the role of the state during pandemics that have had a large impact on societies. After outlining the increasing importance of the World Health Organization (WHO) in dealing with pandemics, we consider why time has proven that the WHO is not a pivotal player in shaping how states respond, resulting in states largely going it alone. Nevertheless, to date, there has been no firm policy conceptualization that has guided states to fully deal with pandemics.

In the second part, we develop the typology of the four phases of policy responses. Here we highlight the importance of anticipating the virus, containing it, controlling it, and then opening up society. This theoretical classification highlights that while there is a sequential, linear flow between the four policy phases, there is also a 'feedback' mechanism at play. This means that while states may be at the fourth phase to pursue policies to 'open up', theoretically they may have to re-install lockdown policies associated with controlling the virus found in Phase 3. This, as we will discuss, was exactly what took place during COVID-19 during the second (and some cases third) waves found in various

https://doi.org/10.1515/9783110743609-004

jurisdictions, which was in part a consequence of the variants of the virus that developed as the pandemic continued.

Modern states, the WHO, and need for policy guidance

Scholars have highlighted the importance of the modern state in trying to deal with pandemics and procedures to be followed, well since the plague. As discussed in Chapter 2, 'an epidemic is generally considered to be an unexpected, widespread rise in disease incidence at a given time. A pandemic is best thought of as a very large epidemic', while TB, Malaria, HIV/AIDS that affect millions yearly are 'persistent pandemics' (McMillen, 2016, 1).

We have already seen in Chapter 2 some historical details of some of the best known pandemics, but what about the policies that were formulated to contain them? Since the plague, even rudimentary policies were developed by the state to deal with pandemics (Delanty, 2021, 7). This includes the 'quarantine and isolation of both people and goods, travel restrictions, prohibitions on public gatherings such as religious assemblies and a general increase of state power over the individual lives of the sick and suspected sick' (McMillen, 2016, 19). Similarly, XIX century cholera 'led to national wide efforts at quarantine' that could only be done by a central state, demonstrating a 'growing association between a state's ability to govern and its ability to keep people free from epidemics' (McMillen, 2016, 5, 20).

Although states realized that they must lead with policies that deal with economic and 'travel' fallouts, along with other policies, there was no firm playbook regarding what they ought to do, and when. De Waal (2020, 22) explains that '(m)ost of the public health measures to deal with cholera began as hand me downs from the medieval plagues, revised during the previous sixty years during the visitation of cholera, adapted each time based on a rule-of-thumb empirical assessment of what had worked and what hadn't.' This rather piecemeal approach was pursued, despite the large impact of pandemics on health and economies. We consider both of these dimensions in turn.

On the first dimension, the impact in terms of raw numbers of death is almost stupefying looking at the plague alone: when it came to Europe in 1347 it eventually took half of the continent's population (McMillen, 2016, 9). Cholera witnessed seven pandemics and it has been estimated that between 21,000 and 143,000 died worldwide of this infection (Ali et al., 2015). Influenza witnessed two waves in 1918, and a third wave in 1919, seeing well over 50 million deaths (McMillen, 2016, 89). HIV/AIDS has now killed 30 million and infected 75 million worldwide (McMillen, 2016, 104). COVID-19 which was declared a pandemic in

March 2020 saw over 3 million deaths reported by April 2021, where the US alone accounted for around a fifth of those.[1]

With regard to the second dimension, historical and recent examples show that epidemics and pandemics can have a huge economic impact. As seen in Yamey et al.'s work (2017, 742), GDP losses associated with the H1N1 Influenza (1918) were 3% in Australia; 15%, Canada; 17%, the UK; and 11%, US. More recently, SARS (2003), witnessed a global economic loss of over USD 52 billion.

Given the impact on these two dimensions, coupled with the lack of guidance that states faced during these health emergencies, there is no surprise that more global, centralized efforts were made to deal with pandemics, led by the WHO. The genesis of this organization stems from world leaders' realization post-Spanish flu in 1918 that 'international health is a problem that demands international cooperation' (de Waal, 2020, 43). When the UN was formed in 1945, the first efforts were thus made by states to set up a global health organization. The WHO was founded three years later in April 1948, with the broad mandate to deal with 'global governance of health and disease... (with) its core global functions of establishing, monitoring and enforcing international norms and standards, and coordinating multiple actors toward common goals' (Ruger and Yach, 2009, 1).

Years after its failed attempt to eradicate malaria in the 1950s (McMillen, 2016, 54), the WHO would eventually gain a pivotal role after SARS in 2003. It did so by developing the 2005 International Health Regulations (IHR) that were shaped by the SARS outbreak. These regulations 'delineate(d) the responsibilities of individual countries and the leadership role of the WHO in declaring and managing a public health emergency of international concern' (Fineberg, 2014, 1335). The 2009 H1N1 pandemic represented a 'test case' for the 2005 IHR, that is, an event that could have solidified the WHO's leadership role in dealing with key pandemics post-2005. However, the 2009 experience resulted in the WHO losing legitimacy, based on lack of transparency within the organization. As Fineberg (2014, 1340) argues, 'the WHO kept confidential the identities of emergency-committee members convened under the provisions of the IHR... (which) fostered suspicions about WHO decision making, which were exacerbated by the failure to apply systemic and open procedures for disclosing, recognizing and managing conflicts of interest.' The effect of this was to reinforce national autonomy in dealing with health crises: this lack of legitimate, global leadership meant that the world was not in a position to respond to health emer-

---

[1] Based on data found on https://coronavirus.jhu.edu/map.html: on April 22, 2021 the total number of global deaths reported was 3,059,018, where the US saw 569,402.

gencies in the 2010s with a unified voice, resulting in domestic level governments dealing with them in a fractured manner.[2]

Consequently, as Horton (2020, 37) explains, without the WHO having a leading role, '... when SARS-CoV-2 arrived there was no global leadership, no willingness to cooperate, and no ability to view what was taking place as a lethal global challenge demanding a coordinated global response. Instead there was inattention, rivalry and accusation.' It was even perceived as being slow to declare COVID-19 a global health emergency: the WHO announced the COVID-19 pandemic on March 11, 2020, where its Director General since 2017, Dr. Tedros, expressed concern about '... the alarming levels of spread and severity, and by the alarming levels of inaction' (WHO, 2020). This, despite some health experts criticizing '... that the novel coronavirus technically qualified as a pandemic weeks before the WHO officially declared it as one, simply because of the wide geographical spread of the cases ...' (Yiu et al., 2020, 9).[3]

Whether or not the WHO's timing on announcing COVID-19 was right, its role was destined to be limited because '... the current IHR (2005) institutional framework is inadequate to cope with some categories of epidemic outbreaks, especially illnesses with high transmissibility and relatively high level of severity' (Yiu et al., 2020, 14). The lack of WHO leadership reinforced the absence of a globally coordinated action in dealing with COVID-19, resulting in national administrations largely acting alone without a precise plan or blue-print of policies to pursue.

The literature (and the experience of citizens worldwide) highlights that these state reactions, particularly in the early part of the COVID-19 pandemic, were wanting and in need of guidance. For example, when US President Trump infamously said in August 2020 that 'the book' was being followed with regard to testing in the US, to which the reporter asked 'what book?', this reflected not only one of the few bizarre comments by the US President, but also the lack of knowledge in what policies should have been followed.[4] Still, while many states did not fully know what to do, there was certainly policy learning from other jurisdictions. For example, Mintrom and O'Connor (2020) ex-

---

2 It is interesting to note that some scholars have argued that the primary role of the state in dealing with health issues was subsequently delegated by states to citizens themselves. As de Waal (2020, 39) notes, '... in the later twentieth century, as chronic, noninfectious, and 'lifestyle' disease took over from infectious diseases as the main threats to health in industrialized countries, responsibility was shifted from states to citizens'.

3 See also McKeever, 2020.

4 Interview with reporter Jonathan Swan (Axios/HBO) in August 2020, see: https://www.you tube.com/watch?v=NmrEfQG6pIg)

amine developments at the state level in the US, showing many governments relied on policy narratives when making policies to deal with the pandemic.[5] Nevertheless, despite some policy learning, many citizens living through COVID-19
would agree with Horton (2020, 86–7) who highlights that there was 'state neg-
ligence' and 'gross incompetence', particularly in the first phase of the disease.

While we do not fully disagree with Horton, we would argue that more than
states having been 'negligent' and 'incompetent,' they were all simply 'ill-ad-
vised' and 'ignorant' – they did not know what needed to be done, why, and
when during a health crisis emergency. In other words, they had no firm, big-pic-
ture policy roadmap, or typology, to follow in the face of uncertainty during a
pandemic. The next section thus develops this roadmap.

The typology: conceptualizing public policy responses in a pandemic

This section develops a theoretical classification scheme of domestic-level policy
phases during a pandemic. This typology, a term which we use conterminously
with 'a classification scheme,' serves as a blueprint for countries developing
public policies when there is no immediate rapid scientific solution with a vaccine or antiviral. Our typology's goal is to offer a roadmap for governments during a pandemic, something that has been lacking to date: while there may be a
scientific solution by the end of the pandemic, our model, '... rejects the wishful
thinking that holds out for a simple fix, such as a vaccine at the beginning of it'
(Dean 2020, 155).

Before developing a typology of the different phases of public policy for
states to follow during a pandemic, it is useful to note from the outset that theoretical classification is common in natural and social sciences: typologies are
essential analytical tools that help us conceptualize, order and comprehend (Collier et al., 2012). For example, natural scientists studying chemistry rely on the
periodic table in order to better understand common traits in certain elements:

---

5 As Mintrom and O'Connor (2020, 206) explain: '...(p)olicy narratives can be thought of as the
general story-lines that emerge and come to hold prominence in policy communities concerning
particular phenomena. An especially important feature of policy narratives is how they can condition the thoughts and actions of broader populations. Those thoughts and actions can, and
usually do, have material consequences for the effectiveness of policies. For example, efforts
to restrict or ban specific behaviors will typically only be effective if they are viewed as consistent with prevailing social norms. That means policymakers seeking conformity with a specific
policy must strive to achieve alignment between the goals of a policy and social norms.'

all carbon-related elements have four electrons in their valence shell, oxygen-related elements two valence electrons and so forth. Our own previous work has developed different ideal-type typologies in social science, where we have theoretically classified different types of policies found in the EU (Chari and Kritzinger, 2006), different types of firms found after privatization (Chari 2015), and different types of lobbying regulatory environments found worldwide (Chari et al., 2010/2019).

As we have argued elsewhere,

> classification schemes will inevitably be debated and challenged: ideal types of systems, as discussed by authors such as Max Weber, are conceptualized based on characteristics and elements of a given phenomenon, but they are not necessarily meant to correspond to all of the characteristics of any one particular case. Nevertheless, a classification scheme serves as a basis for helping us understand common trends as well as differences, even if the concomitant conceptual apparatus does open up some debate (Chari et al., 2019, 178).

Our conceptualization of high/medium/low regulatory lobbying environments, for example, has served as a blueprint for some states to develop their own lobbying laws.[6] Equally important, the subsequent literature on lobbying regulation that followed the typology's development drove science forward by criticizing and building on our work (see, for example, McKay, 2020).

Our conceptualization considers 4 main phases during a pandemic:
- *Phase 1: Anticipating and early virus detection*
- *Phase 2: Containment strategies*
- *Phase 3: Policies to control and mitigate the spread of the virus*
- *Phase 4: Policies aimed at opening up society.*

The first three of these phases are based on initial conceptualizations discussed by the WHO (2018). It highlighted the need for early detection as well as strategies to contain, control and mitigate the virus. This guidance for pandemic preparedness was a consequence of the WHO Review Committee that examined the inadequacies of the 2005 IHR during the 2009 H1N1 pandemic (Fineberg, 2014, 1341). While the WHO's guidance is significant, it suffers two shortcomings. First, the exact policies within the first three phases were not concretely outlined. Secondly, there was no clear path regarding what was required when opening-up society, or what was to be done when the virus potentially re-emerged thereafter.

---

6 See for example the report from the UK's Political and Constitutional Reform Committee (2013), which relies on our regulating lobbying typology in its analysis.

Our typology therefore seeks to build on the WHO's work by outlining key public policy initiatives in all phases, including opening up society, and considering dynamics should the virus remerge after the opening up phase. The following discussion thus considers four dimensions for each of the four phases:

- what is done in the phase;
- when does the phase take place;
- why is it important to do; and
- what public policies would states be expected to pursue in the phase.

This last dimension is vitally important in our typology because it reflects the 'tool chest' states should 'pick from' to respond. In this regard, from a theoretical point of view of policy scholars, we can consider public policies as tools, or instruments, that states have at their disposal to deal with emergencies (Offe, 2021, 31; Dunlop et al., 2020, 368). In the discussion below, we justify the policy instruments found in our conceptualization by consolidating key ideas from the literature from various disciplines.

Conceptualizing and developing the four phases is important for at least two reasons. First, it helps guide states with some certainty so they know what to do in the next pandemic or public health emergency, a guide that was absent during COVID-19. A complete roadmap also offers a blueprint to inform governments what needs to be done as the pandemic (even the one they may now be in) continues. As we will demonstrate later, states may find themselves in second and subsequent waves of a pandemic, and our typology provides a 'feedback mechanism' to help guide them through this.

Secondly, having a typology beforehand shows states the myriad of policies that need to be pursued, decreasing the uncertainty of the multiple policy dimensions they need to act in. This ranges from healthcare, economic, social, regulatory, as well as science and technology policies. Seeing how all may interplay in the various phases gives political actors, civil servants and citizens a 'holistic' view of policies that are expected, when, and why.

We now consider the first phase in more detail, turning to subsequent ones thereafter.

Phase 1: Anticipating and early virus detection

Figure 3.1 offers an initial overview of Phase 1 considering what is done, when is it done, why it is important, and what policies are expected to be pursued.

Anticipation and early detection take place during the epidemic stage of the emergence of virus. In this phase, the main objective is that states pursue poli-

---

1. Anticipating and Early Detection

What is done? State pursues strategies to focus on the threat and early detection to minimize impact

When is it done? Takes place during the epidemic stage of emergence of virus

Why is it important to do? It will save lives and minimize negative impacts (such as economic, and social) that follow in subsequent phases

What policies are expected?

– Develop an Initial Emergency Action Plan (IMAP) to anticipate and detect the threat

– Pursuing regulatory polices of restricting/monitoring movements on international borders

– Start with public information campaigns

Figure 3.1: Overview of Phase 1 of our typology.

cies to focus on the threat and early detection, in order to minimize the short-, medium- and long-term impact. The previous identification of the pathogen would have ideally taken place in order for cogent early detection (de Waal, 2020, 24), but if that is not possible, states have to ensure that part of their initial reaction is to ensure it is done in line with the likely guidance of the WHO. This phase is vital because it will save time (and lives), allowing states to simply implement and/or adapt to the particular pathogenic effect. In their examination of Ebola, the Harvard-London School of Hygiene & Tropical Medicine Independent Panel on the Global Response to Ebola highlighted the importance of acting early, stating that one of the key problems was that 'the long-delayed and problematic international response to the outbreak resulted in needless suffering and death, social and economic havoc, and a loss of confidence in national and global institutions' (Moon et al., 2015, 2207).

We now consider the policies that are expected to be pursued in this phase. It is important to note at the outset, as with all other phases discussed in this chapter, that this is an 'ideal' list of policies that are theoretically expected to be pursued based on international experience during a variety of pandemics and learned best practice. As we will see in Chapter 4 that examines which policies were formulated by different states, some countries may have pursued some policies more than others during COVID-19.

The first, relatively large policy is for the state to define the problem and develop initial plans to deal with the health emergency. Focussing on Canada, Blouin Genest et al. (2021) neatly outline the need to have initial pandemic emergency plans in light of recent health crises, even though they may not always work as governments are not able to adopt their responses quickly in federal states with two levels of governance. They show that in the wake of Mad Cow disease, SARS1 and H1N1 '… countries and subnational entities refined their policy infrastructure to better respond to outbreaks, leading to pandemic emergency plans…' Of course, translating policy into practice may be problematic under emergency conditions; but having a plan still offers guidance of early steps, that can help reduce, if not eliminate, transmission (Hendy et al., 2021, 2).

Building on this literature, we argue that states must develop what we refer to as an **I**nitial **E**mergency **A**ction **P**lan (IMAP) to offer guidance throughout the various stages of the pandemic. In particular, Mazy and Richardson (2020, 562, 569) outline the importance of having a plan and embarking on anticipatory policymaking where governments conduct 'detailed advanced planning … (which) requires a lot of deliberation…'. In our conceptualization, an IMAP, or preparedness plan, may be a complete one, ideally considering what needs to be done based on past experience as seen in all four phases of the typology we develop in this chapter. But at the very least it should include two related dimensions, where the first regards anticipation and the second, early detection.

On the first dimension, an IMAP must recognize the problem, identify the drivers 'that will worsen the impact or facilitate the spread', and isolate/notify high risk patients that may be at more risk of serious illness (WHO, 2018, 29). For example, in the case of COVID-19 at-risk groups included: those over 70, those having a long-term medical condition (such as heart disease or diabetes), and those who have a compromised immune system (immunosuppressed), potentially caused by factors such as cancer treatment, treatment of autoimmune diseases (such as Multiple Sclerosis), HIV, or having an organ transplant.

On the other dimension, an IMAP must outline strategies to coordinate, protect and train healthcare workers to recognize the potential disease, detect it early, and report it immediately (WHO, 2018, 29, 32). Included in achieving these goals is developing plans for emergency investment in healthcare, particularly to train and protect healthcare workers. With regard to protection, this may include the 'facilitation of production of personal protective equipment (PPE), including masks and hand sanitizer and their rapid transparent supply' and the use of diagnostic tests (Shin and Ju, 2020, 279).[7] Protecting healthcare workers is essential as early detection itself 'begins at the health care setting' (WHO, 2018, 29).

A second key policy expected during Phase 1 is pursuing regulatory polices of monitoring and/or restricting movements on international borders. As Hossain et al. (2020, 7) discuss

> We have learnt from the previous SARS outbreak that it is crucial to implement rapid infection control measures to limit the impact of epidemics, both in terms of preventing more casualties and shortening the epidemic period. Delaying the implementation of (border) control measures by 1 week would have nearly tripled the epidemic size and would have increased the expected epidemic duration by 4 weeks... . Previous studies showed that control measures at international cross-borders and screening at borders are influential in mitigating the spread of infectious diseases....

In examination of data during the early phase of COVID-19, they argue that intensive border control resulted in gaining ten days in delaying the spread of the virus (Hossain et al., 2020). This measure was almost immediately taken in Vietnam during COVID-19. As initial cases came from China, the Vietnamese authorities started with policies such as 'screening procedures and mandatory health declarations by passengers, isolation of suspected cases, and eventually complete bans on flights to and from Wuhan and other affected areas' (Hartley et al., 2021, 3).

Interestingly, the evidence on monitoring/restricting movements in the early phases of COVID-19 was brushed off by the WHO. From the last week of January 2020 (when the WHO had declared the public health emergency) until the first week of February, the WHO's Dr. Tedros not only opposed any restrictions for travel against China, but also 'maintained that border closure actions imposed by some member states are an overreaction and not buttressed by science and evidence' (Yiu et al., 2020, 7).

A final set of policies expected to be taken by states in the first phase is to outreach to the public and start with public information campaigns, explaining in a transparent manner key ideas discussed in the previous chapter:
- what the infectious disease threat is,
- how it is transmitted (or, likely transmitted if the threat is novel),
- what its incubation period is (or, estimated period if the pathogen is unknown),

---

7 This may also include securing access to critical supplies of key goods such as respiratory ventilators (Seccareccia & Rochon, 2020). See also Capano (2020).

– and what the first symptoms of having it are.

Experts communicating knowledge and risk ultimately help to educate the public about the pandemic based on facts right from the beginning, which can help minimize misinformation as the pandemic continues (Davis, 2019). Moon et al. (2015, 2209) underline that it is important that 'governments report disease outbreaks early' and in this context they discuss how the 'WHO publicly challenged China's Government to be more transparent about SARS.' Part of this campaign should also see states ensuring that the public is aware of its initial plans to deal with the pandemic, ultimately empowering citizens to feel part of the solution, increase levels of trust, and help determine that the country will successfully overcome the public health emergency (Pandey and Saxena, 2020; McConnell, 2010; Crepaz and Arikan, 2021).

We now consider policies during Phase 2, when the first cases are detected within the territory and there is a need to contain the virus.

Phase 2: Policies to contain the virus

In this phase the state will pursue strategies aimed at effective and rapid containment of the virus as the country experiences its first cases emerging. These steps prevent the pathogen from spreading for as long as possible, taking place during the epidemic stage of localized transmission. The literature shows that countries that acted early fare better in terms of cases, underlining the importance of early containment policies (Migone, 2020a, 272). In this regard, Phase 2 of the typology is important because once it is clear that the virus has arrived in the territory, policies need to be proactively pursued to stop the spread from increasing. We now consider the main policies to be implemented during this phase (we will not repeat ideas on continuing with controlling international borders as these have been raised in our previous discussion of Phase 1).

A first main set of policies is to embark on testing to identify early cases, establishing who the infected person has been in contact with, and if necessary, isolation of infected patients. Historically, this has been seen in various epidemics. For example, in containing SARS, the WHO deemed that 'case isolation, and quarantine of contacts are the most effective control measures' (Crawford, 2018, 41). In dealing with Ebola, key measures included 'rapid identification and isolation of cases with strict barrier nursing' (Crawford, 2018, 36), tracing patient contacts, 21-day quarantine and public engagement by addressing issues such as funerals. These ideas of 'testing, tracing, and isolation' were oftentimes ex-

---

2. Strategies to Contain the Virus

What is done? Policies towards effective and rapid containment as the first cases are detected

When is it done? Takes place during the stage of localized transmission

Why this is important? Policies need to be proactively pursued to stop/retard the initial spread of the infection within the territory

What policies are expected?

– Testing, contact tracing and isolation

– Ensure Healthcare infrastructure in place with increased investment

– Continue with information campaign, to minimize 'infodemic'

– Continued restricting of international borders

– Starting initiatives to promote R&D

Figure 3.2: Overview of Phase 2 of our typology.

pressed during COVID-19 (see: Dean 2020, 151; Horton, 2020, 71), but it is worth looking at the importance of these in some detail.

On testing, Kelly-Cirino et al. (2019, 6) highlight that historical outbreaks of Ebola, Lassa fever, yellow fever and Zika viruses '... have been exacerbated by the lack of accessible diagnostic tests, lending to poor detection and surveillance, ultimately delaying the time to containment.' In this regard, they argue that 'diagnostic tests are a fundamental component of a successful outbreak containment strategy, being involved at every stage of an outbreak, from initial detection to eventual resolution' (Kelly-Cirino et al., 2019, 1). Unfortunately, to this day tests do not exist for several diseases such as Crimean-Congo haemorrhagic fever, Nipah and henipaviral diseases, and Rift Valley fever. Where they do exist, for diseases such as SARS, Zika Virus Disease, and Filoviruses (Ebola and Marburg), and most recently COVID-19, it is because they received international focus and funding, crucial to develop critical diagnostics.

The reasons that not only early testing, but also continuous testing throughout a pandemic are crucial is because they can save thousands of lives during the containment of the outbreak and billions of dollars later on (with lockdown policies discussed in Phase 3). As Kelly-Cirino et al. (2019, 1) explain on its immediate impact:

> poor diagnostic preparedness has contributed to significant delays in the identification of recent outbreaks for multiple pathogens, including Ebola, Lassa fever, yellow fever, and

> Zika.... in the 2013 – 2016 Ebola epidemic in West Africa, there was a 3-month delay between the index case and the identification of the causative agent; postoutbreak analyses suggest that diagnosing 60 % of patients within 1 day instead of 5 days could have reduced the attack rate from 80 % to nearly 0 %

Importantly, even when a vaccine may be developed (as conceptualized in Phase 4 of our typology discussed later), continuous testing is essential. This was seen during the yellow fever outbreak in Central Africa in 2016 – 17 where

> ... there was a severe shortage of reagents, meaning that laboratories were unable to carry out tests on the majority of suspected cases.... (causing) significant delays in recognizing the outbreak, hindering the roll-out of the vaccination programme and diminishing the effectiveness of target vaccination, resulting in increased spread of the disease and longer time to containment (Kelly-Cirino et al., 2019, 3).

Once identification of those testing positive is made, health authorities can try to trace those who have been in close contact with them to ascertain who else may have been at risk of infection. In the case of COVID-19, close contact meant more than 15 minutes of face to face contact within 2 meters of someone infected, however this time period was significantly shortened with the highly transmissible delta variant. As Hendy et al. (2021, S88) discuss in the case of New Zealand during COVID-19 'contact tracers in regional public health units interviewed confirmed and probable cases about their contacts during their infectious period, which is usually considered to be up to 2 days prior to symptom onset.' This was reflective of developments in states throughout the world including South Korea which received praise for their early efforts (Di Moia, 2020, 657). It is important to note that testing and contact tracing of asymptomatic cases is also important as seen in COVID-19: while a person may not be showing symptoms, they may still pass it on to others, particularly those who may be from at-risk groups.

Initial measures to test and trace go hand in hand with those to prevent spreading within the community, specifically isolation and quarantine. While the terms are oftentimes used coterminously, there are technically slight differences between them, succinctly defined by the US Department of Health and Human Services as follows:

– **Isolation** separates sick people with a contagious disease from people who are not sick.
– **Quarantine** separates and restricts the movement of people who were exposed to a contagious disease to see if they become sick. These people

may have been exposed to a disease and do not know it, or they may have the disease but do not show symptoms.[8]

Hartley et al.'s (2021, 4) examination of Vietnam during the beginning of COVID-19 show that its '… intensive contact-tracing and quarantine efforts were triggered to contain the spread.' COVID-19 saw cases of quarantine for all who may have been infected, as seen in the early stage of the spread of COVID-19 when the Diamond Princess cruise ship in Yokohoma was quarantined, turning 'the ship into a floating petri dish' as described by Honigsbaum (2020, 274).[9]

A second set of policies includes making sure there are enough resources targeted towards healthcare. In this regard, if Phase 1 saw that plans for increased investment for healthcare were being made, Phase 2 sees this plan coming into full motion. Studies on COVID-19 have shown that having robust healthcare systems are important. For example, Vera-Valdés (2021, 269) considers 23 explanatory variables on health, political and economic factors to ascertain their impact on the number of cases and deaths during COVID-19, where one of their main findings is that 'hospital beds per thousand inhabitants are a statistically significant factor in reducing the number of deaths.' Cifuentes-Faura (2021, 246–7) gives examples of expenditure that increased in different EU states during COVID-19, including: Germany, where additional health care expenditure was around EUR 19 billion; Italy, 845 million for personnel and purchase of medical devices; and Spain, 1 billion for infrastructure and 2.8 billion for regional transfers (as Spain's healthcare is implemented at the regional level; see Chari and Heywood, 2009). State investment would also go towards personal protective equipment for healthcare workers, which, if not regulated well, would result in the public buying into this to the chagrin of those that really need it (Addo et al., 2020; see also Horton, 2020, 44).

The third policy countries should pursue is dealing with an 'infodemic', which refers to 'rumours, gossip and unreliable information' (WHO, 2018, 34). While states must inform the public of the pandemic during Phase 1, in Phase 2 states must deal with mass publics receiving too much information that may

---

8 Taken from: https://www.hhs.gov/answers/public-health-and-safety/what-is-the-difference-between-isolation-and-quarantine/index.html

9 Quarantine can also be applied to those coming in from other countries. This was seen in South Korea during the start of COVID-19: while the government did not ban outright travel from China, they introduced strict quarantine measures: '… President Moon announced that the government would not ban Chinese entry. Instead, he said it would strive hard to minimize the risks by strengthening quarantine policy in cooperation with the Chinese government' (Lee et al., 2020, 372).

or may not be accurate, making it hard for them to find trustable sources and cogent guidance.[10] De Waal's work on Ebola (2020, 46) shows the impact on how people being exposed to correct information can make a difference: both communities and epidemiologists learn to think alike. When turning to COVID-19, Horton (2020, 38–9) discusses different dimensions of an infodemic, including: 'conflicting theories about the cause of the disease... the symptoms of the illness and how the virus is transmitted... alleged Covid-19 cures... and (propagating) misinformation deliberately aimed to deceive.' False information may be transmitted in the news, or stories that are deliberately intended to deceive readers. The latter was especially salient during COVID-19 in Facebook and WhatsApp, where Sloan (2020, 195) examines how this disease represented a first social media infodemic helping contribute to an overabundance of unreliable information.

A fourth key initiative countries should pursue during the second phase is to promote Research and Development (R&D) to find a vaccine and/or antiviral solution. While policies to spur R&D start in Phase 2, they continue throughout the next phases of the pandemic to find a solution to end the disease. Underlying the importance of science and technology policy and the need to pursue R&D, Honigsbaum (2020, 273) laments that 'prior to ... SARS (2003), coronavirus research was considered a dead end' and thereafter 'has been a victim of boom and bust funding' despite SARS and MERS-CoV (2012).

Given this boom and bust nature of funding, it is important that public bodies – not private actors – play a primary role in:

> ...manufacturing, research, and development for drugs, vaccines, diagnostics, and other non-pharmaceutical supplies (such as personal protective equipment) where the commercial market does not offer appropriate incentives. For known pathogens... (this includes) invest(ing) in bringing candidate drugs, vaccines, technology platforms, and other relevant products through proof of concept, phase 1, and phase 2 testing in humans, so that they are ready for wider testing, manufacturing, and distribution when an outbreak strikes... (As the disease progresses during an outbreak this would include mobilizing) finance for priority research and development projects, such as diagnostics for novel pathogens (Moon et al., 2015, 2214).[11]

The reason why the state has to play a key role in R&D is because private actors have generally failed to see the vaccine market in particular as lucrative. Monrad et al. (2021, 2) highlight that:

---

10 WHO Situation Report 13, February 2020.
11 See also Yamey et al. (2017, 742) who highlight the importance of global investment in R&D.

private investment in infectious disease vaccines too often falls far short of what would be the socially optimal level, compared to other biomedical products... vaccine sales rarely constitute a large share of revenues for leading pharmaceutical producers. This problem is exacerbated in the case of pathogens primarily affecting populations in lower-income countries with less purchasing power... where a sustained demand for the vaccine is not guaranteed and investments are particularly risky from a commercial purpose.

Given that vaccine development may not be lucrative for pharmaceuticals, a means to incentivize them to complete the costly three phases of trials is to embark on Advance Purchase Commitments (APCs), as took place for COVID-19 candidates. These 'work by having the funder (i.e. the state) pre-commit to purchasing doses of a vaccine, conditional on it being successfully licenced and produced' (Monrad, 2021, 2).

However, there are two theoretical problems with APCs, from both pharma companies' and a government's perspective:

-   Firms may be hesitant to sign APCs. If an epidemic is small, fewer doses would be needed, and therefore the renumeration that a pharmaceutical receives would be small (Monrad et al. 2021, 2). So, from a business perspective it may actually be advantageous for a firm to delay signing an APC and develop a vaccine only when there is a large, global outbreak.
    Even in a global outbreak, the benefits for a firm developing a vaccine may be mixed.
    -   On the one hand, a firm may not benefit as much as one would have expected. For example, while Pfizer and AstraZeneca developed two of the most administered vaccines globally during COVID-19, their stock market increases were 12.4% and 7.3% respectively between June 8, 2020 (when the vaccines were being developed) and June 7, 2021 (when the global rollout was taking place).[12] While this may seem like a good increase within a year, it actually pales in comparison to other listed companies that increased much more in the same time period, including Netflix (17.9%), Microsoft (34.8%) and Apple (51%).
    -   On the other hand, a firm may be very successful. For example, in some contrast to Pfizer and AstraZeneca, the relatively smaller and newer company Moderna that was formed in 2010, which commercialized a mRNA vaccine against COVID-19 as mentioned in Chapter 2, saw its stock price increase by over 271%.

---

12 The stock market data used to analyze developments in the US market (between June 8, 2020, and June 7, 2021) for all the companies mentioned in this sub-section were found on https://www.bloomberg.com/markets/stocks

- Countries may be counting on deals that pharmaceuticals eventually renege on. This may impact the rollout of the vaccine in certain political systems, as seen in Europe during COVID-19 which we discuss in Phase 4 (the Opening Up Phase) below.

We now consider policies during Phase 3, when a surge in the number of cases is detected within the territory and there is a need to mitigate the spread.

Phase 3: Policies to control and mitigate the spread of the virus

In this phase, the state will pursue policies to control and mitigate the virus's spread as the case numbers surge. Taking place during the epidemic stage of amplification, the policies pursued will reduce the mortality rates, and the long-term impact of the pandemic to the economy and society.

The start of this phase will be marked with an initial surge in the number of cases, meaning a sharp or sudden rise in cases followed by either sustained, or exponential growth. Before we consider ways that a surge may be measured, it is important to note something policy makers should be cognizant of: there are measurement errors which may make it difficult for states to draw a clear line when one phase ends and another starts, pointing to the importance of the reliability of data (Lipsitch, 2020, 92). For example, when trying to measure the start of Phase 2 (when the first cases arise) and when Phase 3 starts (when there is a start in the surge of the number of cases), states may not necessarily have complete data to ascertain this. Numbers may be inaccurate because the virus could have been circulating without being counted and cases may not have been recorded given lack of diagnostic tests or people seeking treatment. Especially at the start of COVID-19, we saw these errors because '(w)hen a person is exposed to the coronavirus, it can take up to two weeks before they become sick enough to go to the doctor, get tested and have their case counted in the data.'[13] In this regard, it is important that policy makers prioritize obtaining solid data to inform policies pursued (Ioannidis, 2020, 103).

Assuming there is access to reliable data, how can we measure the start of a surge that marks the beginning of Phase 3? A key way of measuring this is to consider when the 'surge' into the Intensive Care Unit (ICU) starts. Considering

---

13 https://www.hopkinsmedicine.org/health/conditions-and-diseases/coronavirus/first-and-second-waves-of-coronavirus

3. Policies to Control and Mitigate the Virus' Spread

What is done? Strategies to control and mitigate the impact as cases surge: reduce mortality and disruptions to economy and society

When is it done? Takes place during the stage of amplification

Why is it important? Policies need to be pursued to deal with the severe health, economic and social impact on society during this phase

What policies are expected?

- Lockdown policies, including: closing schools, working/restricting movement from home, internal and international travel bans, restrict public events and gatherings
- Economic policies to deal with: job losses, household relief, economic stimulus
- Healthcare: Testing, contact tracing, universal access to treatment
- Social policies: human rights protection; preventing evictions from homes; countering increasing racism & domestic abuse; addressing mental health challenges; problems in long-term care homes, meat packing facilities, and high infection areas
- Policies to spur R&D

Figure 3.3: Overview of Phase 3 of our typology.

Ireland as an example, after the first case of COVID-19 came to public attention on February 29, 2020, the Health Protection Surveillance Centre (HPSC) stated that the 'surge' into ICU started to happen in Epidemiological Week 11, March 8–14; this saw six cases, whose number started to rise rapidly after so that by Epidemiological Week 12 (March 15–21) there were 31 ICU cases.[14]

In the absence of ICU data, or given that those with the disease may not necessarily be admitted into the ICU, another proxy for measuring the start of surge is to consider the evolution of daily new confirmed cases numbers: the start of a surge is evident when there is a marked increase in the 7-day rolling average, that is followed by a sustained increase in cases over time that may be potentially exponential. Looking at the data for Ireland in Graph 3.1, a marked increase in

---

14 See: https://www.hpsc.ie/. We are indebted to Dr. Catherine Hayes of Trinity College Dublin, School of Medicine, for insights on this.

the number of cases that is followed by strong positive growth is seen after March 12, which is similar to the start of surge as measured by looking at ICU data as explained above.

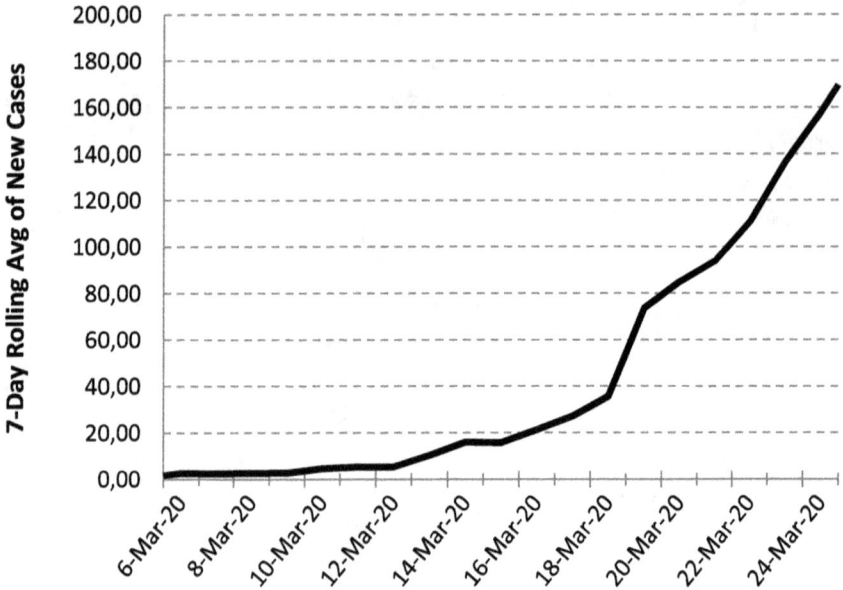

Graph 3.1: Daily new confirmed cases in Ireland (rolling 7-day average), March 2020. Source of data: https://ourworldindata.org/

In terms of Phase 3's importance, this is the epidemic stage that has the most significant impact on citizens' health given the sheer number of cases and deaths that may occur as the infectious disease amplifies. This is by far the most difficult phase for states to deal with, as they need to find a balance between:

(a) seeking to control the virus spread by way of restrictive control measures and
(b) dealing with negative consequences in society in doing (a).

In other words, on the one hand, 'lockdown' policies need to be pursued to mitigate and control the virus as its spread amplifies, with the aim to flatten the number of cases and lower mortality (Anderson et al., 2020). On the other, these policies need to be tempered with key economic and social policies to counter the negative impact of lockdown.

Turning to the first set of policy tools states have at their disposal in Phase 3, what is meant by 'lockdown' policies? The myriad of lockdown policies that countries may pursue include: closing childcare facilities, as well as moving primary, second-level, and third-level educational facilities 'online'; restricting movement within a certain limit from home; work from home orders; closure of non-essentials shops; restricting public events and gatherings; and travel bans both internally as well as internationally (Hale et al., 2020; Hartley et al., 2021 4, 6; Devakumur et al., 2020; Fong et al., 2020; Blum and Dobrotić, 2020; El Masri and Sabzalieva, 2020; Carpenter and Dunn, 2020). The timing to pursue lockdown is important because the longer it is delayed as cases surge, the higher the death toll with a highly contagious infectious disease that is easily passed in the absence of physical distancing between people. This is demonstrated by Balmford et al.'s (2020, 525) epidemiological models across eight countries during COVID-19 that demonstrate that 'a further week long delay in imposing lockdown would likely have cost more than half a million lives. Furthermore, those countries which acted more promptly saved substantially more lives than those that delayed.'

However, governments face a trade-off between saving lives and short-term economic impact: early lockdown sees higher financial and economic impact on society, even though more lives are saved; later lockdown sees a lesser cost to the economy, while more lives are lost (Balmford et al., 2020, 537). While Balmford et al.'s (2020, 546) investigation concludes that early lockdown may be hard but it creates a net benefit to society by saving a large number of lives, the COVID-19 pandemic saw states such as the US and Brazil acting relatively late when pursuing lockdown (as discussed more fully in the next chapter.)

It is worth noting the difficulties in implementing lockdown, and the paradoxes sometimes found within lockdown policies. With regard to implementation, the COVID-19 experience shows that expecting street level bureaucrats to implement some of these measures did not come without its problems, especially for those like police. This is seen in Davidovitz et al.'s (2020, 1) investigation on Israel that shows that additional duties for essential workers enforcing the regulations resulted in 'increased policy ambiguity, higher risk exposure, and expanded discretion.'

Contradictions between lockdown policies can also be seen when we consider potential dynamics regarding internal and international border control. Wood et al.'s (2007) examination of Australia shows that internal border control is effective in delaying the spread of a pandemic within a county. To this end COVID-19 witnessed several states not allowing travel between regions, especially those experiencing outbreaks. However, Europe witnessed inconsistent policies with regard to both internal and international travel as COVID-19 continued. As an example, during March 2021 local travel within France (say, between Paris and Marseille) was not allowed, but travel between France and Spain (say, between Paris and Madrid) was. This effectively allowed for many French to bizarrely take vacations in Spain, even though they were not allowed to move within their own country. This shows that the harmonized approach that could have taken place in the EU, effectively did not.

A second set of policy tools tackle the financial downturn brought about with lockdown. These 'economic policies' include those to provide income support for those on the labour market (such as pandemic unemployment payments, or temporary wage subsidy schemes)[15] and financial and fiscal support for businesses. These incentives have been prominent in many states during COVID-19 and investigated by scholars. For example Stylianou (2021, 2) examines developments in Australia and notes that it 'responded to the pandemic by providing A\$259 billion in fiscal and balance sheet support to business (equivalent to 13.3 percent of annual GDP)', and highlights that 'wage subsidy schemes' were implemented in various countries. Attempting to assess the effectiveness of these initiatives, Madeira's (2020) investigation on Chile examines tax relief measures and direct income and expenses support, arguing that tax measures had a limited impact when compared to support actions that were relatively stronger. In the case of the EU, it is important to note that funding of economic policies came from national treasuries as well as the supranational level of governance. Ladi and Tsarouhas (2020, 1048) show how in the summer of 2020 the EU saw the negotiation of the 'Recovery and Resilience Facility (RRF), with €310 billion in grants envisaged to be dispersed to member states'. This highlights how with COVID-19 the EU took on an increasing 'redistributive function', transcending its historical regulatory role associated with big policy areas such as single market, competition policy, and economic and monetary union (Majone, 2014).

Healthcare policies constitute a third set of policy instruments in Phase 3. While we have examined testing, contact tracing and isolation in the previous phase, these become even more problematic to implement well as case numbers rise. Plümper and Neumayer (2020, 17) argue that as cases surged during COVID-19 'test, trace and isolate was dead in the water as a strategy given the sheer flood of infections before it even properly started to take off....'

Also, countries need to critically ensure in this phase universal access to treatment as healthcare facilities reach 'surge capacity' with increasing cases and volume of patients (Yanzhong, 2009). This includes developing strategies:

---

15 Goldmann (2020, 1298) considers policies such as labour market support during a pandemic to be akin to basic 'human rights'.

to enhance bed capacity '... to accommodate the surge of more critical patients into the acute areas'; to train and enhance personnel response to care, for example, 'for a large number of ventilated patients'; and to consider the use of alternative care facilities 'to alleviate incoming surge at hospitals' (Phillips, 2006, 1104). The WHO emphasized the need for universal coverage by stating that countries should 'ensure that everyone, especially the most vulnerable, can access the essential health services they need without experiencing financial hardship.'[16] As the UN Office of the High Commissioner of Human Rights highlights,

> ... people in vulnerable situations who are often neglected from health services, goods and facilities, include(e) those living in poverty, women, indigenous peoples, people with disabilities, older persons, minority communities, internally displaced people, persons in overcrowded settings and in residential institutions, people in detention, homeless persons, migrants and refugees, people who use drugs, LGBT and gender diverse persons. Many of them may have lived experience of poverty and find themselves in situations where they are most likely to be exposed to the risk of contagion, yet the least likely to be protected from COVID-19 or supported by adequate and timely tests and health services.[17]

With this in mind, a final related set of policies during Phase 3 are denominated as 'social policies' which are expected to deal with the negative consequences of lockdown (Fuller, 2020, 112; Dean 2020, 149). Key policies that governments may need to develop include: ensuring that human rights are protected, especially amongst those such as the homeless; preventing evictions from homes as well as rent increases for those hit hard economically by the pandemic; countering increasing racism, as took place during COVID-19 against the Asian community particularly in North America; and addressing mental health challenges, including depression and increases in suicide (Klingberg, 2020; Berkowitz et al., 2020; Li and Galea, 2020; Park, 2021; Wilson et al., 2020, 617; Parsell et al., 2020). Another key policy includes dealing with escalating domestic violence during the pandemic, where COVID-19 saw countries pursuing domestic violence reduction strategies (Soremi and Dogo, 2021; Ertan et al., 2020). Finally, states may need to address problems in crowded spaces (such as long-term care homes, meat packing facilities) where there is high severity or harmfulness of the disease (virulence) as seen during COVID-19. To this end, Béland and Marier (2020) examine developments in Canada, especially seen in the tragedy in Québec at the start of

---

16 Taken from https://www.who.int/news-room/feature-stories/detail/governments-push-for-universal-health-coverage-as-covid-19-continues-to-devastate-communities-and-economies
17 See: https://www.ohchr.org/EN/NewsEvents/Pages/DisplayNews.aspx?NewsID=26484&LangID=E

the pandemic when several seniors died in nursing homes, where there was a clear need to develop better long-term care policies.

We now consider policies during Phase 4, when society opens up after successful mitigation and control of the virus.

Phase 4: Policies aimed at opening up society and eradicating the virus

This phase takes place during the epidemic stage of reduced transmission of the virus. The main objective is to make a successful transition from the mitigation phase towards pre-viral status quo, ensuring the eradication of the virus. This is important because 'opening up' is crucial for the re-establishment of stability in the economy and society. However, opening up too quickly may result in a return to the amplification of the virus, when there is a second or subsequent wave of the virus. This means that states may have to revert to pursuing Phase 3 (lockdown) policies.

In terms of the overarching goal expected in Phase 4, states formulate policies to ease restrictions pursued in Phase 3. This will take place in a phased basis when there is a clear evidence that it is safe to do so. The main indicator in this regard will be the suppression, and ideally the eradication, of the number of cases of those with the disease. This is determined with continuous testing and contact tracing as took place in the previous phases.

Ideally the state would have developed a flexible 'Roadmap' for opening up, outlining the gradual lifting of Phase 3 lockdown policies, as well as formulating measures to re-establish employment and the economic system to the pre-pandemic status quo. This 'lifting lockdown' needs to be clearly communicated to the public in order to minimize misunderstandings, and even 'stigma' that may emerge.[18]

As seen with COVID-19, it is also vital that states anticipate contingency plans in case the viral threat needs to be mitigated again. This will take place when there is a second or subsequent waves of the pandemic. Having waves of pandemics is nothing new, as seen in Influenza pandemic in 1918 and 1919.

The case of COVID-19 similarly saw the velocity of new waves emerging within in a short period of time, oftentimes with increasing force. Using data from Ire-

---

[18] In terms of clear communication, Hargreaves & Logie (2020, 1917) 'suggest three policy priorities to minimise potential increases in COVID-19 stigma (during lockdown lifting): limit fear by strengthening risk communication, engage communities to reduce the emergence of blaming, and emphasise social justice to reduce judgement.'

> **4. Opening-up Society and Eradicating the Virus**
>
> *What is done?* Strategies to open up society after the mitigation phase to reach the pre-viral status quo
>
> *When is it done?* Takes place during the stage of reduced transmission
>
> *Why important?* Opening up is crucial for re-establishment of stability in the economy and society.
>
> *What policies are expected?*
>
> – Roadmap for lifting Phase 3 lockdown restrictions on a timed basis, and re-establishing the economic system
> – Continuous testing and contact tracing
> – Contingency plans in case viral threat needs to be mitigated again with a second (and subsequent) wave(s) of pandemic (feedback with Phase 3)
> – Best Practice for Vaccine/Antiviral Rollout: transparency, safety, universal access, consistency
> – Policies to continue to spur R&D (including investigating variants/strains of virus)

Figure 3.4: Overview of Phase 4 of our typology.

land as an example, Graph 3.2 helps demonstrate how clearly waves were seen in some states during COVID-19, underlining the importance of having contingency plans.

In Graph 3.2 we see that the seven-day rolling average of daily new confirmed cases saw three waves: the first with a peak around mid-April 2020; a second, with a peak in the third week of October; and the final wave peaked slightly before mid-January 2021.

This demonstrates the potential push and pull of moving in the typology, demonstrating a type of 'feedback' states face in having to oscillate between Phases 3 and 4 when there are waves:

– Wave 1: As the spread of the virus amplified in from early March, and throughout April 2020 during the first wave, Phase 3 policies were pursued to mitigate the virus as discussed in more detail in Chapter 3. This resulted in a drop in case numbers.
– Wave 2: Phase 4 opening-up occurred thereafter, and the subsequent number of cases that ensued was worse than the first. Almost cyclically, this second

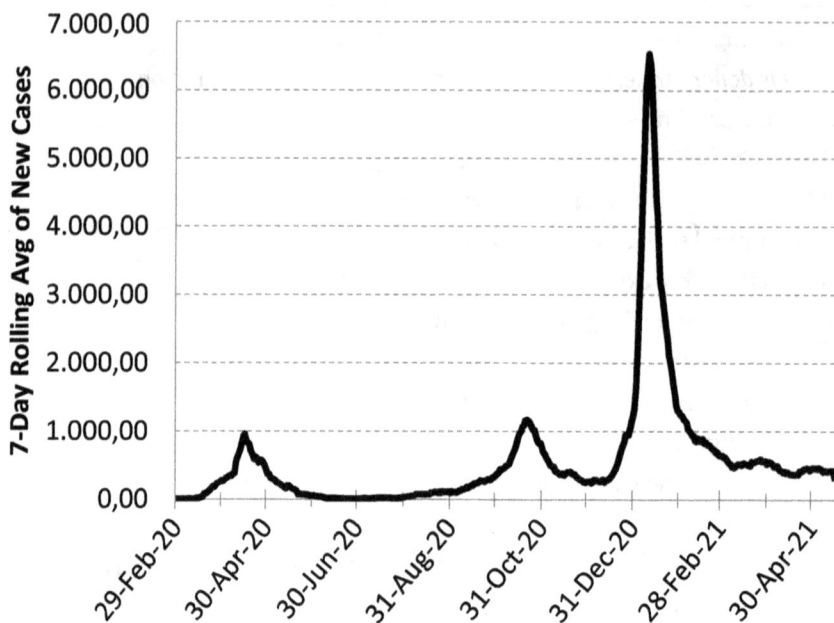

Graph 3.2: The three waves of COVID-19 in Ireland: 7-day rolling average of confirmed cases between March 2020 and May 2021. Source of data: https://ourworldindata.org/

   wave was again countered with Phase 3 policies, then a relaxing of those policies as Opening up (Phase 4) was again attempted in early December 2020.

– Wave 3: the opening up was yet again met with subsequent surge of cases between the end of December and early January 2021, when there was a third wave. This was even worse than the second wave, primarily due to the UK variant (alpha) of COVID-19 that was rampant in Ireland. This resulted in a return to Phase 3 policies of lockdown, which lasted effectively well into May 2021 for fear of a fourth wave.

While COVID-19 did see the development of a vaccine solution in a short amount of time, many pandemics do not see a rapid vaccine or antiviral solution as discussed in Chapter 2. Even only very recently, when we consider the history of pandemics, did we see that smallpox vaccination was considered a 'monumental public health achievement' (McMillen, 2016, 40); to this day, vaccines do not exist for pandemics such as AIDS, even though great advances have been made in terms of anti-HIV treatments. Having vaccine or antiviral solutions arrived at theoretically allows for an opening up, but five key, interrelated steps need to be taken, including some of which were previously explained in Chapter 2:

1. A transparent and robust drug/vaccine approval process by regulatory authorities (e. g. FDA or EMA)
2. Post-marketing surveillance
3. Securing access to the vaccines/antivirals, including negotiating APCs, prompt delivery and universal distribution amongst all of the population
4. Transparent information campaign during the rollout
5. A consistent, clearly articulated rollout plan

The worldwide experience of the COVID-19 rollout shows that following/implementing all of these five steps is not simple; we will consider each in turn.

First, the 3-phased approval process for vaccine development (discussed in Chapter 2) was done in an incredibly short amount of time by several regulatory authorities globally during COVID-19, ensuring safety, efficacy and quality. However, the regulatory approval process was seen with different 'speeds' globally, and even within some continents. Looking at Europe alone, we saw that the UK's Medicines and Healthcare products Regulatory Agency (MHRA) approved the Pfizer vaccine on December 2, 2020, while the European Medical Agency (EMA) approved it weeks later on December 21.[19]

Second, when states needed to proactively monitor the safety of the vaccines once approved, we saw during COVID-19 that some vaccines were temporarily paused or suspended (in the cases of AstraZeneca and Johnson & Johnson). This was because both vaccines were associated with development of rare blood clots.[20] Regulatory authorities, like the FDA, acted with an abundance of caution as seen in the Johnson & Johnson rollout by monitoring the situation, temporarily suspending it, and attempting not to lose the public's confidence in the vaccine.[21]

Third, several countries throughout the world – as well as the political system of the EU which acted on behalf of its 27 member states – secured access to the COVID-19 vaccines by signing advanced purchase commitments (APCs) with several pharmaceuticals. One major hiccup, however, was seen in January 2021

---

19 For the press release on the UK, see: https://www.gov.uk/government/news/uk-medicines-regulator-gives-approval-for-first-uk-covid-19-vaccine; on the EU, see: https://www.ema.europa.eu/en/news/ema-recommends-first-covid-19-vaccine-authorisation-eu#:~:text=EMA%20has%20recommended%20granting%20a,from%2016%20years%20of%20age

20 See https://www.bbc.com/news/world-us-canada-56733715)

21 For the Joint FDA DCD press release can be found here: https://www.fda.gov/news-events/press-announcements/joint-cdc-and-fda-statement-johnson-johnson-covid-19-vaccine when the EU upheld that AstraZeneca did not respect their APC as it was sending fewer doses than negotiated, thereby slowing down the rollout process.[22] In April 2021, the EU even launched legal action against AstraZeneca for its failure to meet delivery and contractual agreements.[23]

More worrying from a global perspective is the inequality between high, medium and low income states regarding the number of doses purchased from pharmaceutical companies: as of mid-April 2021, rich countries fared well in securing vaccine treatments, while poorer ones where most of the world lives lagged well behind (Graph 3.3).

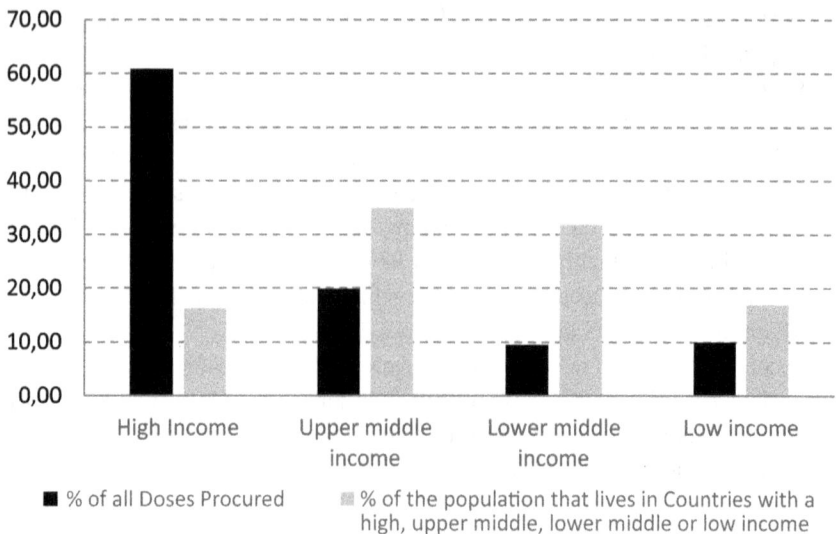

Graph 3.3: Advanced COVID-19 doses purchased globally: % of vaccine doses purchased by country income and % of the population that lives with a high/upper middle/lower middle/ low income. Sources: Elaboration of data from Duke Global Health Innovation Center and World Bank (as of 16/4/21).

Graph 3.3 shows that the 4.7 billion doses procured in high income countries was 3 times higher than that in upper middle income countries and 6 times that

---

22 On Pfizer and the EU, see: https://www.ft.com/content/59a014d0-aacc-43a5-b061-8ea4b25c3c00. On a full list of APCs the EU negotiated see, https://ec.europa.eu/commission/presscorner/detail/en/qanda_20_2467
23 See: https://www.reuters.com/world/uk/eu-preparing-legal-case-against-astrazeneca-over-vaccine-shortfalls-politico-2021-04-22/

of lower middle and low income (black columns).[24] This, despite these high income states representing only a fraction (less than 20%) of the total population sampled (light grey).[25] As Duke's Global Health Innovation Center states: 'Many high-income countries have hedged their bets by advance purchasing enough doses to vaccinate their population several times over.'[26]

Fourth, turning to information transparency during the rollout, states must strive for high trust amongst the population about vaccines by ensuring that citizens have full knowledge about them. Publishing their findings in December 2020 (before the full rollout of COVID-19 vaccines), Paul et al.'s study over 32,000 adults in the UK interestingly shows the following:

> Distrustful attitudes towards vaccination were higher amongst individuals from ethnic minority backgrounds, with lower levels of education, lower annual income, poor knowledge of COVID-19, and poor compliance with government COVID-19 guidelines. Overall, 14% of respondents reported unwillingness to receive a vaccine for COVID-19, whilst 23% were unsure. The largest predictors of both COVID-19 vaccine uncertainty and refusal were low-income groups (< £16,000, a year), having not received a flu vaccine last year, poor adherence to COVID-19 government guidelines, female gender, and living with children. Amongst vaccine attitudes, intermediate to high levels of mistrust of vaccine benefit and concerns about future unforeseen side effects were the most important determinants of both uncertainty and unwillingness to vaccinate against COVID-19. (Paul et al., 2021, 1)[27]

While the COVID-19 rollout did initially see many uptake the vaccine in early 2021, doubts increased globally with fears that the AstraZeneca and Johnson &

---

24 There are over 150 countries in this sample established by the Duke Global Health Innovation Center, corresponding to the following: *1. High Income Countries:* Australia, Canada, Chile, Croatia, Cyprus, member states of the EU-27, Hong Kong, Israel, Japan, Kuwait, Macao, New Zealand, Oman, Panama, Qatar, San Marino, Saudi Arabia, Singapore, South Korea, Switzerland, Taiwan, The United Kingdom, United Arab Emirates, Uruguay & The United States of America. *2. Upper Middle Income:* Albania, Argentina, Azerbaijan, Belarus, Bosnia, Brazil, China, Colombia, Costa Rica, Dominican Republic, Ecuador, Indonesia, Iran, Iraq, Jordan, Kazakhstan, Lebanon, Malaysia, Mexico, North Macedonia, Paraguay, Peru, Serbia, South Africa, Thailand, Turkey & Venezuela. *3. Lower Middle Income:* Algeria, Bangladesh, Bolivia, Cambodia, Egypt, El Salvador, Honduras, India, Morocco, Myanmar, Nepal, Pakistan, Palestine, The Philippines, Senegal, Sri Lanka, Tunisia, Ukraine, Uzbekistan, Vietnam & Zimbabwe. *4. Lower Income:* countries of the African Union. Source of Doses Procured, Duke Global Health Innovation Center, Data from April 16, 2021, available at: https://launchandscalefaster.org/covid-19/vaccineprocurement.
25 Data to calculate the population in the sample of countries across the income levels is from the World Bank (2019), at https://data.worldbank.org/indicator/SP.POP.TOTL
26 Quote taken from: https://launchandscalefaster.org/covid-19/vaccineprocurement
27 See also Priori et al. (2021) that similarly show that there was hesitancy amongst some the population to take the vaccines during COVID-19.

Johnson vaccines were associated with blood clots.[28] This was tempered by politicians, health regulators, and firms alike emphasizing that vaccines were safe despite this 'very rare event'.[29]

Fifth, states must have consistent plans on the rollout process itself – once a plan is carefully drafted, it is important to stick to it. Of course, it may be necessary to change the timing of the plan if vaccines are not available, as happened with many states when the Johnson & Johnson vaccine was temporarily suspended during COVD-19. However, a prime example of an inconsistent plan is when the government says it will vaccinate the population in a certain order, and then changes plans midway. This was seen in Ireland during the COVID-19 rollout when the state reneged on an initial plan that prioritized teachers be vaccinated.[30]

As a final policy goal in Phase 4, it is important to note that R&D remains crucial and a vital part of any state's response when opening up, even during a vaccine rollout: while Phases 2 and 3 of our typology emphasized the importance of funding to find a solution to the disease, R&D remains essential in Phase 4 on two grounds. First, there are some parts of the population that may not be able to take a vaccine as discussed in Chapter 2, and antiviral drug development funded by the state may be the only solution for them.

Second, even with a vaccine, R&D with regard to investigating variants/ strains of virus and developing solutions needs to continue. As discussed in Chapter 2, there are several variants of the SARS-CoV-2 virus that causes COVID-19, ranging from those originating in the UK (alpha), South Africa (beta), Japan/Brazil (gamma), and India (delta). The CDC denominates these as 'variants of concern' (VOCs), meaning that they showed evidence of increased transmissibility and disease severity as well as 'reduced effectiveness of treatments or vaccines, or diagnostic detection failures.'[31] This suggests that R&D

---

28 See: https://www.nytimes.com/2021/04/14/world/europe/western-vaccines-africa-hesitancy. html

29 See: https://www.irishtimes.com/news/world/fauci-johnson-johnson-vaccine-blood-clots-a-very-rare-event-1.4536518

30 When the vaccine rollout plan in Ireland was first developed in early 2021, there was a promise to vaccinate teachers in order to convince teachers that they could safely go back to work in primary and secondary schools. But, the government later reneged on this once schools opened, developing instead a revised plan vaccinating by different age groups only (i.e. not based on occupation) once healthcare workers, those over 70, and the medically vulnerable received the jab. For more information, see: https://www.irishtimes.com/news/ireland/irish-news/teach ers-warn-vaccination-changes-undermine-efforts-to-keep-schools-open-1.4524266

31 https://www.cdc.gov/coronavirus/2019-ncov/cases-updates/variant-surveillance/variant-info.html#Concern

must be pursued to continuously test the efficacy of existing treatments given the emergence of variants.

Synthesizing the phases – the typology

Taking the four phases together, Figure 3.5 offers the typology of policy responses during a pandemic.

The versatility of the typology is that it can be used by anyone to better understand developments in any state, anytime, during any pandemic when there is no immediate vaccine or antiviral solution. And even where there is a treatment, the model conceptualizes best practice in eradicating the virus. Thus, the classification scheme offers not only a foundation from which future scholarship can build, but also a roadmap to guide states developing policies during various phases.

Four broad points of the model stand out.

- While the model linearly flows from Phases 1–4 (seen with the top arrow), it incorporates a feedback mechanism to account for a second and any subsequent wave (conceptualized with the feed-back arrow at the bottom). This may occur when policies of opening up fail and policies to control and mitigate need to be reinstated, as we saw during COVID-19 in 2020 and 2021.
- Each country may have different dates for the start and ending of the different phases, some of which may be seen more than once if there are second and third waves. So, there is a time-specificity that guides our understanding of developments in any country, accounting for variations in the phase that different countries may find themselves in at any one time. For example, on the same date the United States may find itself in Phase 4, while India may be in Phase 3.
- Our typology takes into consideration what governments do as case numbers increase or decrease, thereby allowing them to take 'political action' informed by empirical based, scientific observations (Fuller, 2020, 111). As the typology also outlines what strategies need to be pursued when the first cases arise, it is even theoretically possible that if policies to contain the virus in Phase 2 are done well then states may not even need to enter into Phase 3.
- Regardless of whether or not there is feedback, some policies can be found in more than one phase, as seen with strategies towards international border restrictions as well as R&D. This highlights the importance of multiple dimensions of policy, some of which may be part of a country's toolbox throughout a public health emergency.

1. Anticipating and Early Detection	2. Strategies to Contain Virus	3. Policies to Control and Mitigate Virus	4. Opening-up Society and Eradicate Virus
Takes place during the epidemic stage of emergence of virus	Takes place during stage of localized transmission	Takes place during stage of amplification	Takes place during stage of reduced transmission
What is done? State pursues strategies to focus on the threat and early detection to minimize impact	*What is done?* Policies towards effective and rapid containment as the first cases are detected	*What is done?* Strategies to mitigate the impact as cases surge: reduce mortality & disruptions to economy and society	*What is done?* Strategies to open up society and reach the pre-viral status quo
What is expected? - Develop an Initial Emergency Action Plan (IMAP) to anticipate and detect the threat - Pursue regulatory polices of restricting and monitoring movements on international borders - Start with public information campaigns	*What is expected?* - Testing, contact tracing and isolation - Ensure healthcare infrastructure in place with increased investment - Continue with information campaigns to minimize 'infodemic' - Continued restricting of international borders - Start initiatives to promote R&D	*What is expected?* - Lockdown policies: closing schools, working/restricting movement from home, internal and international travel bans, restrict public events and gatherings - Economic policies to deal with: job losses, household relief, economic stimulus - Healthcare: Testing, contact tracing, universal access to treatment - Social policies: human rights protection; preventing evictions from homes; countering increasing racism & domestic abuse; problems in long-term care homes, meat packing facilities, & high infection areas - Policies to spur R&D	*What is expected?* - Roadmap for lifting Phase 3 lockdown restrictions on a timed basis, and re-establishing employment and the economic system - Continuous testing and contact tracing - Contingency plans in case viral threat needs to be mitigated again with a 2nd (and subsequent) wave of pandemic (feedback with Phase 2 and 3) - Best Practice for Vaccine/Antiviral Rollout: transparency, safety, universal access, consistency - Policies to continue to spur R&D (including investigating variants/strains of virus)

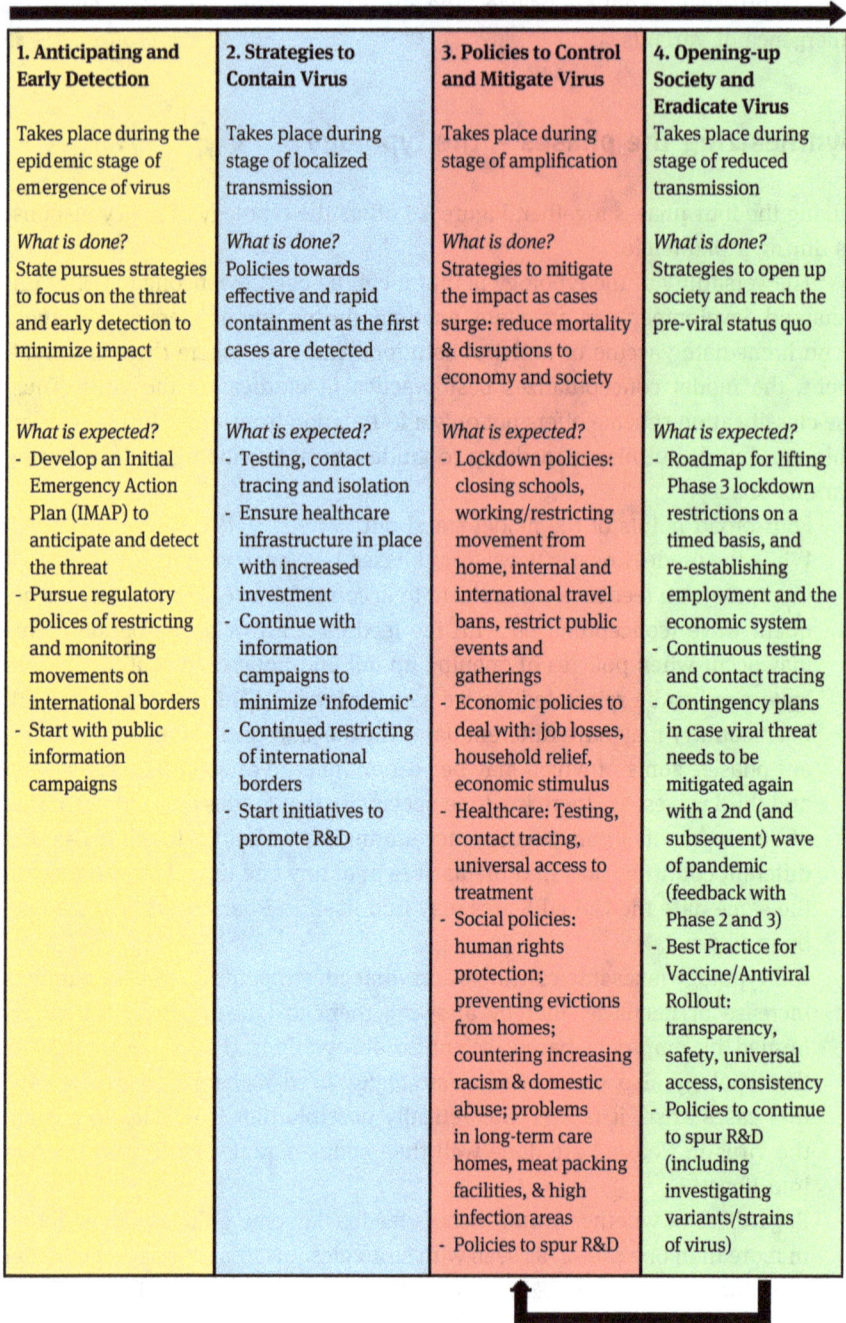

Figure 3.5: The four phases of public policy responses during a pandemic.

Limitations of the typology

Our typology indicates what policies should be pursued by countries based on best practice during the different phases of a pandemic. But, as with any classification system in science, our typology has some limitations.

First, our typology outlines the policies to be formulated by the state, but it is up to each state to decide full details of the policies and, importantly, with which stakeholders to negotiate these details. For example, policies largely denominated as those related to 'health' will see a different plurality of actors involved in formulation, such as doctors, nurses, independent health regulatory agencies (such as the CDC in the US) that will bring their expertise to the policymaking table. Regulatory policies dealing with border closure could involve not just health officials, but also airport regulatory authorities, firms from the aviation sector and unions. In contrast, 'social policies' may involve civil society organizations, NGOs, and even the state's security forces to help shape policies to, for example, mitigate and deal with domestic violence and racism. Public policy scholars for years have highlighted the balancing act between fostering participation amongst different interest groups while creating stability and efficient policies in modern democracies, and this is even more complicated during a health emergency when decisions need to be taken quickly. But it is still important to respect this balance, or run the risk of having a democratic state be accused of being dictatorial.

With this is in mind, some scholars suggest that being in a democracy may actually make one worse off during a pandemic, almost giving the erroneous interpretation that living in a dictatorship can be beneficial for one's health. For example, Cepaluni et al. (2020) argue that '(Covid) policy responses in democracies were less effective in reducing deaths in the early stages of the crisis.... (implying that) democratic political institutions may have a disadvantage in responding quickly to pandemics.'[32] Nevertheless, this finding is countered by other scholars demonstrating that democratic states report cases and death figures more frequently, and are 'more effective at reducing fatalities' (Baris and Peluzzo, 2020, 216)

A second limitation to our typology is that while it offers a broad outline of policies to be formulated, we are cognizant of the different ways the policies may be implemented, or how the policy is rolled out once it has been formulated. Thus, while the typology highlights what needs to be done, there are complexities of how translating the policy's goals into action is done 'well', or how this

---

32 See also Serikbayeva et al. (2020)

could be done 'better', invariably coming with more experience. This is seen with a clear example raised by Dean (2020, 152–3) that shows that contact tracing's implementation ultimately determines the policy's success:

> contact tracing, in particular, relies heavily on the skills of interviewers to earn trust of patients so they feel comfortable sharing important but sensitive information. A successful tracer may have a particular way of structuring an interview, or even use a particular tone of voice. Outside consultants can facilitate but not replace the learning process. Rather than being told what works participants benefit from the discovery process itself – measuring performance, finding the outliers, and seeing firsthand what makes them more effective.

Finally, our typology puts the state and its policy responses at the center of dealing with pandemics. This is akin to intergovernmental scholars of EU politics that see the European integration project driven by member states, not by supranational institutions such as the European Commission (Chari and Kritzinger, 2006, Chapter 3). While international guidance during a pandemic may be found from organizations such as the WHO, a key assumption in our model is that states are the key drivers of formulating the myriad of policies required during a pandemic and the domestic level of governance is thus tasked to formulate policies. This does not mean, however, the framework established in the typology cannot be transposed to a different level of governance. For example, in the future, should the WHO (or the EU) play *the* leading role in developing specific policy responses that are then transposed at the domestic level, the model itself can still be used by these international organizations to inform them of the policies they need to tell states to pursue, when, and why.

Conclusions

The first part of the chapter offered a brief description of the role of states during pandemics, why there has been a lack of global leadership led by the WHO, and the need for firm conceptualization of policies to be pursued by countries during a pandemic. Justifying the components of our classification system based on ideas raised in the literature and best practice, we thus developed the typology of the four phases of policy responses that states need to pursue: anticipating and early detection of the virus, containing it, controlling and mitigating it, and opening up society. The policies found in these phases range from healthcare, economic, social, regulatory, and science and technology. Our typology highlights a linear flow between the four policy phases, but also incorporates a 'feedback' mechanism at play. This shows how states experiencing a second wave may need to reconsider pursuing policies to control and mitigate the virus if the opening up phase sees difficulties.

The classification scheme developed in this chapter offers a roadmap that guides states developing public policies during the various phases of a pandemic, that can be applied by anyone, anywhere, during any pandemic. The next chapter will test the theoretical classification developed in this chapter. By using our model as a backdrop against which to evaluate what was done or not in various states during COVID-19, we provide evidence to better understand how states comparatively performed. As such, our evaluation of countries' experience will illuminate challenges and lessons countries may face in future pandemics.

Chapter 4
Demonstrating the strength of the typology: examining key countries globally

In this chapter we demonstrate the strength of the classification scheme developed in Chapter 3. We do so by comparing the public policies pursued in key countries during the COVID-19 pandemic to the expectations in our typology. These countries are (alphabetically): Canada, Chile, Germany, India, Ireland, New Zealand, South Africa, and the United States. The first section justifies why these states are chosen. The second outlines the methods of analysis used in this chapter, which relies on both qualitative and quantitative methods. The third section, the heart of the chapter, analyzes developments in these countries. We close by offering a comparative overview of the vaccine rollout.

Justifying the countries examined

Deciding which countries to examine with regard to COVID-19 puts comparative public policy scholars in somewhat of a dilemma: examining a large number of say 40 countries prevents nuanced analysis of developments in a single country; while a single country study runs the risk of having too few observations to draw generalizations from. With this in mind, our reasoning behind our country selection was based on two key steps.

As a first step, we examined various data including that of confirmed deaths in countries around the world since April 2020. We were aware, however, that at the start of COVID-19 states may have measured a COVID death differently, where some deaths clearly related to COVID-19 may not have been recorded as such.[1] To minimize this error, we decided to lag our analysis of early deaths in the pandemic by considering the cumulative number by October 2020, which was after over half a year since the WHO declared COVID-19 a pandemic in March 2020.

Thus, in Graph 4.1 the top 45 countries worldwide in terms of cumulative deaths on October 30, 2020 are considered. Countries whose bars are darker on the graph represented those we 'shortlisted' to be examined in more detail for two main reasons. First, was their location across the continuum on the graph, where we see some countries at both ends, as well as in the middle, of

---

1 For example, on India see Pulla (2020).

https://doi.org/10.1515/9783110743609-005

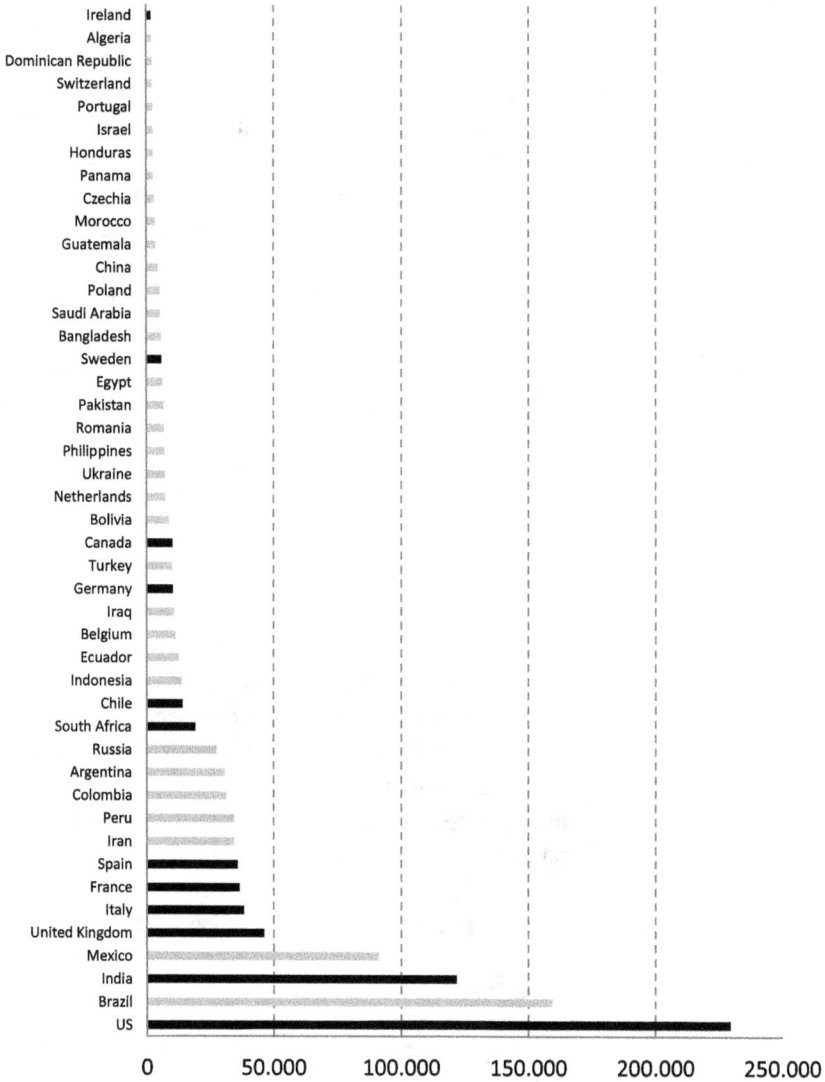

Graph 4.1: Cumulative COVID-19 deaths, October 30, 2020 (Raw Deaths, Top-45 Globally, Oct 30). Black columns indicate those countries shortlisted in a first instance for the present study. Source: Johns Hopkins Corona Virus Resource Center.

the x-axis. Though not on the graph, we also considered New Zealand that had experienced only 25 deaths, one of the lowest in the world at the time. Second, was the countries' geographic location across the world, representative of significant cases across all continents.[2]

In a second step, we took those shortlisted countries and then saw how they compared against each other on a normalized scale, given the limitations of looking solely at the raw numbers of deaths that will be a related to the size of the population. We did so by considering the number of deaths per 100,000 people in the country (Graph 4.2).

Graph 4.2 shows the evolution of normalized values between April 20 and October 30, 2020 on 3–5 days' intervals, allowing us to see similarities and differences in order to come up with a definitive list of countries. Four observations can be made, justifying our final case selection:

–   With its deaths at the lowest value on the graph, investigation of New Zealand allows for insights against states which have seen higher cases/deaths.

–   While Germany is seen closer to the left-hand side of the Graph in 4.1 when compared to Ireland, in Graph 4.2 we see the opposite: by October 2020 Ireland has more deaths than Germany per 100K. Interestingly, the normalized value in Ireland is actually closer to France than it is to Germany, perhaps going against expectations given Ireland's place on Graph 4.1 and the generally accepted view of its solid handling of the crisis.[3]

–   In terms of a noteworthy pairwise comparison based on geographic proximity, we note that the US sees significantly higher normalized values (and steeper positive growth) when compared to Canada, allowing for fruitful evaluation of two bordering states seeing notably different outcomes.

–   In terms of the amplification of the disease, we see exponential growth in the death rate of Chile, which has had one of the highest rates in all of Latin America throughout COVID-19. Exponential growth is also seen in South Af-

---

2 A critical reader will note that a source of error in the data is how countries measure COVID-19 deaths, especially at the beginning of the pandemic: there may be an issue of the reliability of the data. Interestingly, this has historically been an issue as McMillen (2016, 99) argues: 'In Italy, civil authorities forced the country's most influential newspaper, Corriere della Sera, to stop publishing (the influenza) death toll as fear and anxiety mounted.' This is not different to Brazil in June 2020 when Bolsonaro stopped publishing data, only to be instructed by the Supreme Court to do so. While such flagrant examples are not an issue for most states, there was nevertheless, no full agreement between states on a harmonized measure regarding what constituted a COVID-19 death (e. g. only those dying in hospitals, only those dying after a positive infection test had been obtained, etc.).

3 See, for example, the *Globe and Mail*'s report on: https://www.theglobeandmail.com/world/article-leo-varadkar-lauded-for-steady-handling-of-covid-19-crisis-as-ireland/

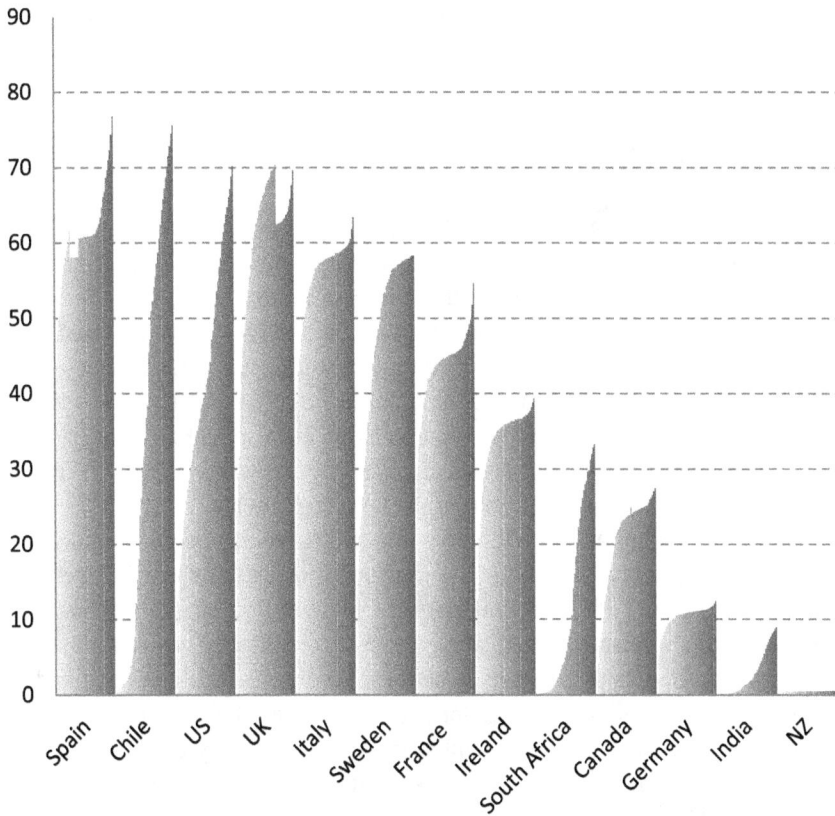

Graph 4.2: COVID-19 deaths per 100,000 evolution in the period between April 20 and October 30, 2020. Source: Johns Hopkins Corona Virus Resource Center.

rica and India, where both have experienced a significant history of pandemics.[4] Given that all are found at different points of Graph 4.2's continuum, investigating them allows for some potentially novel comparative insights.

Considering these observations, this chapter will analyze eight countries across several regions in the world: Oceania (New Zealand), Europe (Ireland and Germany), North America (the US and Canada), South America (Chile), Africa

---

4 India has historically seen cholera, influenza, plague, smallpox and TB, while South Africa has witnessed HIV/AIDS, influenza and TB (Chopera, 2020).

(South Africa) and Asia (India). This allows for a truly global comparison of the policies pursued during COVID-19.[5]

Methods of analysis

To answer how countries responded with regard to the policy expectations found in the various phases of the typology developed in Chapter 3, we rely on a mixed method approach using both qualitative and quantitative methods.

The first, more qualitative, approach relies on analysis of publicly available documents, including reports from government ministries, press releases, and newspaper articles. These were available on government webpages as well as various websites, such as covid19policywatch.org. We also rely on the emerging number of academic articles and book chapters that are written about COVID-19, integrated in our narratives for each of the countries below.

In terms of quantitative analysis, we rely on several databases to attain empirical evidence to establish both the timelines (in terms of which dates the states went into the different phases) and the policies pursued. Regarding when the different phases started, a main source was the Our World in Data database that allowed us to ascertain when the different phases started and ended for each state. This empirical indicator permitted us to see when the first cases arose (start of Phase 2), when the initial surge took place by measuring the 7-day average of cases (start of Phase 3, as discussed in the previous chapter), and when that 7-day average plateaued (start of Phase 4). With regard to the policies pursued, we relied on the data available in the Oxford COVID-19 Government Response Tracker (OxCGRT) database developed by Hale et al. (2020a & b). A final crucial database to better understand restricting/monitoring international borders was the CAPA Centre for Aviation database.[6]

Appendix A offers supplemental information on the book's methods of analysis for this chapter. Here, we outline in more detail how this mixed method approach was used to measure when the Phases started and then to capture the policy responses of the state during the phases. This can be used as a guide

---

5 Some of these states have been researched before by the Research Team, including the US, Canada, Chile, Ireland, and Germany (see Chari et al. 2019; Chari, 2015; Chari and Bernhagen, 2011).

6 Of all the databases utilized in this chapter, this is the only one that is not publicly available. We are indebted Arlene Healy and the Staff at TCD library for securing access to this, as well as Sam Cui from CAPA. More information on it can be found on: https://centreforaviation.com/data/profiles

to replicate this study for other countries beyond even those studied in this book, which will be of particular interest to scholars and policymakers worldwide.

Presentation of findings and visualization of an ideal scenario

In terms of presentation of the country experiences, we have decided to visually portray this using 'timelines', which show the major policies/initiatives that each country formulated during the different phases. We had originally considered presenting tables, but in many cases these extended to well over 3 to 4 pages, which could be difficult for readers to follow. In contrast, the timelines we present offer the reader a neat, succinct summary of the main points which can be easily visualized. Further, the presentation of the timelines is colour coded with the colour scheme established in the previous chapter for each of the phases, which allows for an easy understanding of the main findings.

In terms of expectations, Figure 4.1 considers an 'ideal timeline'. In the bottom part of the figure, below the black arrow, we show the phases and the empirical indicator for the start of each phase. In the top part above the arrow, we show the main policies one would ideally expect to have been pursued as discussed in Chapter 3. So, policies expected in Phase 1 are in yellow; those expected in Phase 2 are in blue; Phase 3 policies are in red; and those in Phase 4, in green.

Figure 4.1 demonstrates what we may analogously call a type of 'layer cake' – all of the policies theoretically found in Phase 1 (in yellow) would be found when the country is in the phase of anticipating the virus before there are cases; Phase 2 policies (in blue), when first cases are found; Phase 3 policies (in red), when there is a clear surge; and Phase 4 policies (in green) when the number of cases have gone down significantly and states can open up.

In contrast, in a non-ideal case we may effectively see a type of 'marble cake' in the timeline, meaning that the colours at the top of the figure are mixed, or out of order. This would be the case, for example, if a country pursues Phase 4 policies of opening up during the time-period that a country is in Phase 3 when it should have formulated policies to control and mitigate. In this example, we would see some green over the top of Phase 3 of the timeline, where theoretically there should have been only red. As we will see, this is exactly what happened in Ireland during the 2nd and 3rd waves.

We now consider the different countries in turn, starting with New Zealand. This is a clear example of a state that has, at the time of writing, controlled the virus better than any major state in the world. We highlight that it is the closest

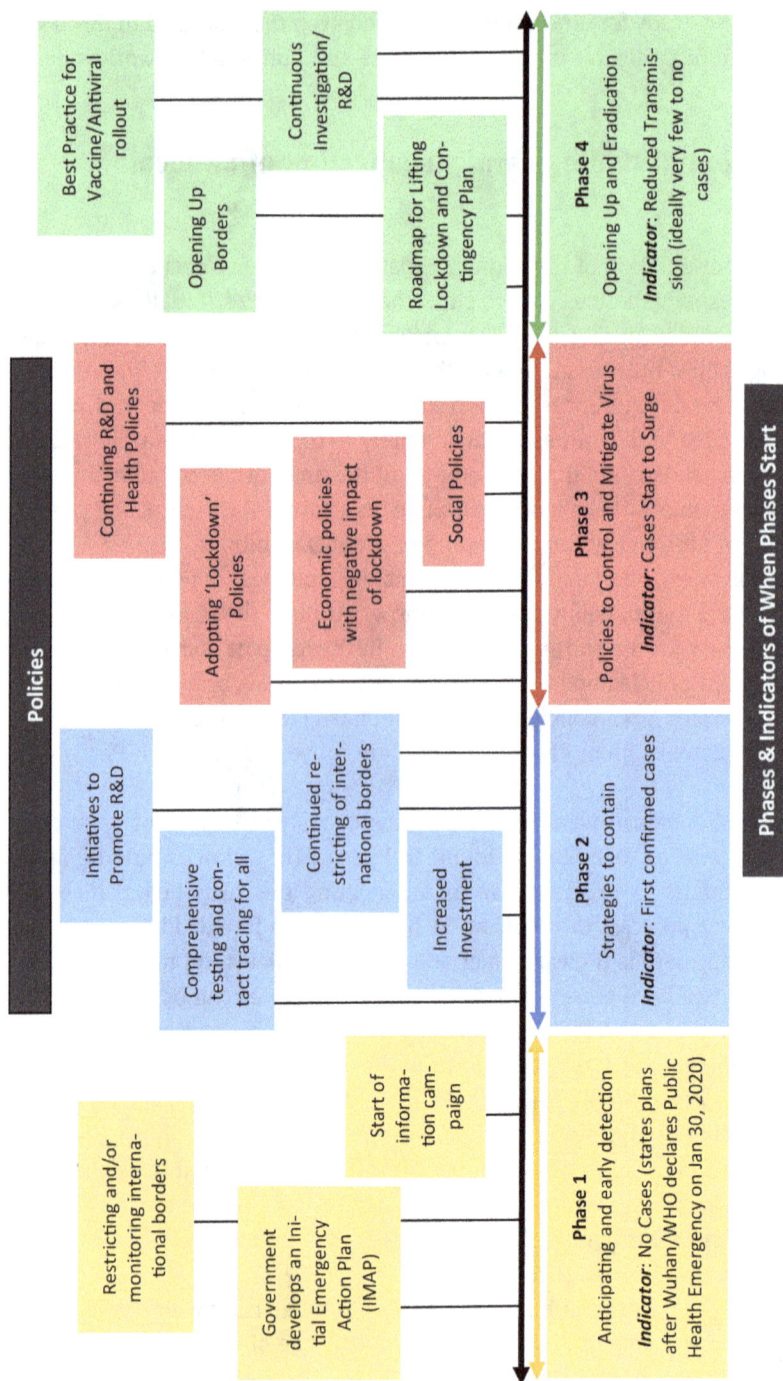

Figure 4.1: Ideal timeline of policies and phases.

example in our study of having attained a timeline that resembles a 'layer cake' as visualized in Figure 4.1.

We then turn to Europe, where attention is paid to the three waves found in Ireland. To compare developments of how other European states dealt more effectively with waves when compared to Ireland, we focus on the policies pursued by Germany.

We then turn to comparative examination of the United States and Canada, the latter of which was able to cope better with COVID-19 when there was no vaccine solution.

We close by comparatively examining developments in those countries that witnessed relatively longer first waves and some of the hardest hit by the pandemic: India, South Africa and Chile.

There are two dimensions to our discussion which the reader should note from the start. First, our main objective of this analysis is to consider how states performed against the expectations in our typology as outlined in the previous chapter. As such, our narrative below does not offer a detailed analysis of all the developments during COVID-19 in each state, which would go well beyond the objectives of this book. However, in giving our short, succinct analysis of how the states fared against the expectations in our typology, we integrate arguments made in key contributions in the literature to date which the reader can turn to for further reading.

Second, our discussion considers the policies during the first wave of the virus, whose length of time interestingly varies as we will see. The exception to this is Ireland (where we show policies during the 1st, 2nd and 3rd waves) and Germany (where their 1st and 2nd wave are examined), highlighting the feedback mechanism of our typology.

New Zealand: keeping the virus at bay

Horton (2020, 71) argues that New Zealand represents an 'astonishing story of success', having experienced fewer than two dozen deaths and fewer than 1500 total cases by mid-May 2020 while the rest of the world was being ravaged with COVID-19. Hendy et al. (2021) highlight that Prime Minister Jacinda Ardern and her team reacted quickly by: restricting borders; pursuing widespread testing, isolation and contract tracing; and eventually triggering a lock down. All of this coupled with 'clear crisis communications' and public information campaigns (Dean, 2020, 150). As Mazey and Richardson (2020, 563) argue, 'the discourse became about eliminating the virus... rather than managing it', which one may argue set it apart from most countries.

This success can be explained because the government relied on specialist expertise, including that from the Director-General of Health Dr. Ashley Bloomfield, and made decisions which were evidence driven: both Ardern who was trusted amongst the population and Bloomfield 'stayed firmly on the same page and completely on message throughout the crisis' (Mazey and Richardson, 2020, 562).

Graph 4.3 considers the rapid rise and fall of COVID-19 in New Zealand by looking at the 7-day rolling average of new cases over time between the end of February and May.

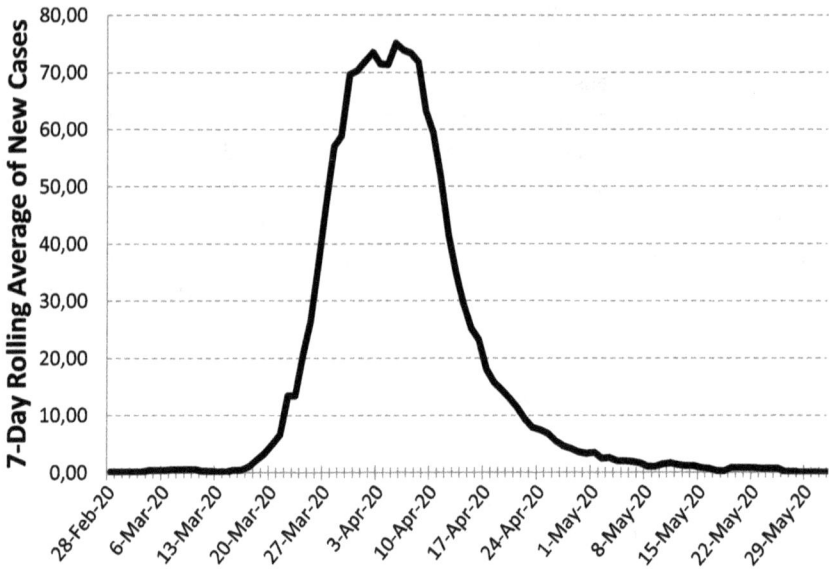

Graph 4.3: New Zealand: 7-day rolling average of new cases February–May 2020. Source of data: https://ourworldindata.org/

We arrived at the dates used in our analysis with regard to when Phases 2, 3 and 4 started by considering the 7-day rolling average as follows:

– Phase 2: This phase starts on February 28, 2020, when the first case was seen.
– Phase 3: The beginning of Phase 3 occurs when cases started to see an initial surge on March 22, where the 7-day average was at 13.42 which was almost twice that from the day before at 6.57. The peak of the wave is found on

April 5, which saw the highest 7-day average at 75 for the time under discussion, plus the highest number of new cases that day at 89.

– Phase 4: The start of Phase 4 is seen by April 28, when the 7-day average had dropped to a little more than 4 and the graph subsequently flattens. There were some slight increases in August 2020, October 2020, and March 2021, which resulted in some local lockdowns as seen in Auckland in August 2020. However, there has not been a second wave in the country as of the time of writing (June 2021), meaning that the last phase was effectively seen at the end of April 2020.

When seeking to gauge how New Zealand fared against our typology, Figure 4.2 visualizes the major policies pursued by the country during the four phases: the top part of the figure that is seen above the black arrow shows the main policies and the dates they were pursued/started, while the bottom part of the figure shows the range of dates for each of the phases as explained above.[7]

Overall, one can argue that of all the countries examined in this book, New Zealand approximates most closely a timeline characterized as a layer cake: it pursued almost all of the policies expected in each of the phases in the typology at the time when they should have been formulated. The only exception is the slight delay in having something similar to a type of Initial Emergency Action Plan (IMAP, as discussed in the previous chapter) that would guide the state on the types of policies/measures to pursue during the pandemic. Ideally, this should have been formulated in Phase 1, before the first cases arrived. The fact that this was not done is reflective of a criticism made in the literature: the country needed 'to be much more anticipatory, rather than reactive, in the approach to policymaking' (Mazey and Richardson, 2020, 566).

Nevertheless, by the end of Phase 2 of our typology New Zealand eventually established their four Alert Levels. These are:

– Level 1, prepare (disease is contained);
– Level 2, reduce (disease is contained but risks of community spreading are growing);
– Level 3, restrict (heightened risk that disease is not contained); and
– Level 4, lockdown (likely that disease is not contained).[8]

---

7 Beyond the main sources outlined in Appendix A and noted in this section, we have also consulted https://www.health.govt.nz/ in the development of our narrative and timeline for New Zealand.

8 See: https://covid19.govt.nz/assets/resources/tables/COVID-19-alert-levels-summary.pdf

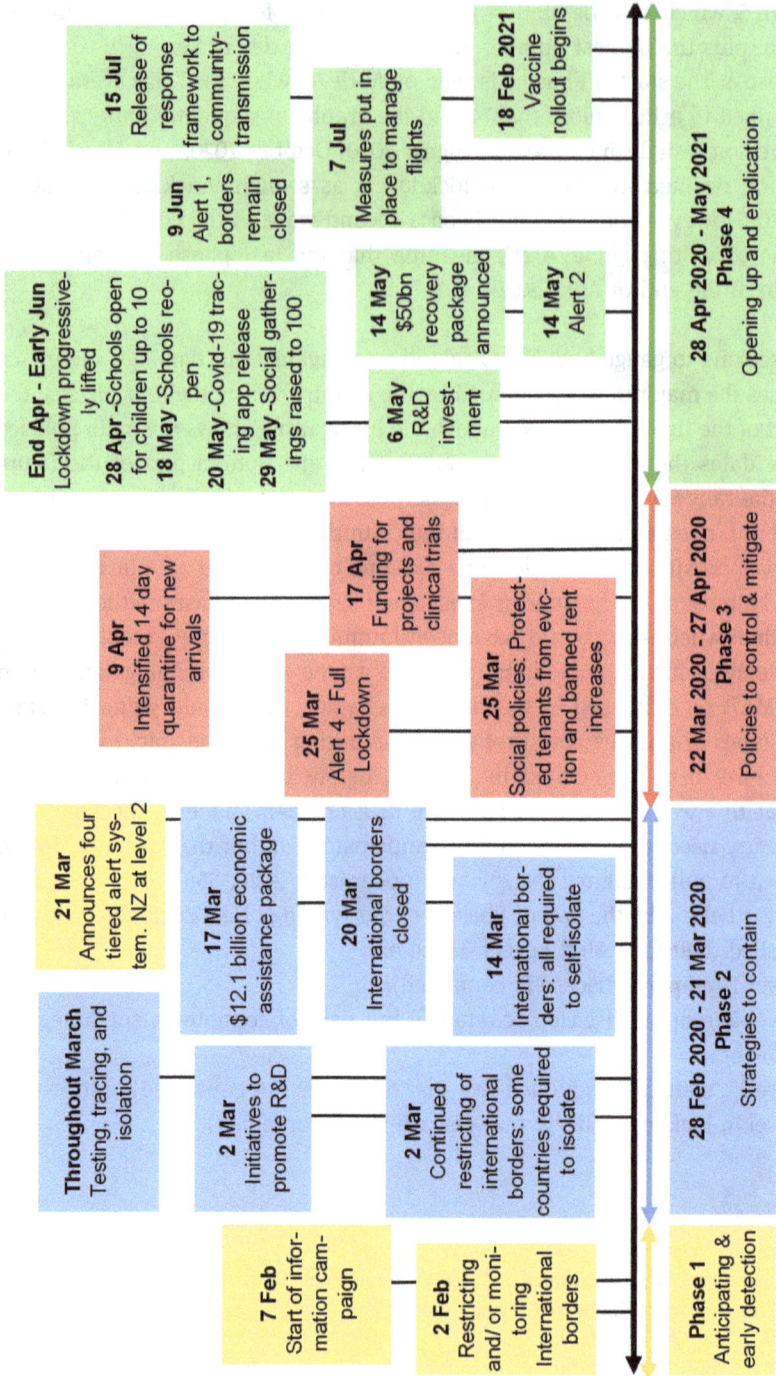

7 Feb Start of information campaign

2 Feb Restricting and/ or monitoring International borders

Throughout March Testing, tracing, and isolation

2 Mar Initiatives to promote R&D

2 Mar Continued restricting of international borders: some countries required to isolate

21 Mar Announces four tiered alert system. NZ at level 2

17 Mar $12.1 billion economic assistance package

20 Mar International borders closed

14 Mar International borders: all required to self-isolate

9 Apr Intensified 14 day quarantine for new arrivals

17 Apr Funding for projects and clinical trials

25 Mar Alert 4 - Full Lockdown

25 Mar Social policies: Protected tenants from eviction and banned rent increases

End Apr - Early Jun Lockdown progressively lifted
28 Apr -Schools open for children up to 10
18 May -Schools reopen
20 May -Covid-19 tracing app release
29 May -Social gatherings raised to 100

9 Jun Alert 1, borders remain closed

6 May R&D investment

14 May $50bn recovery package announced

14 May Alert 2

15 Jul Release of response framework to community-transmission

7 Jul Measures put in place to manage flights

18 Feb 2021 Vaccine rollout begins

Phase 1 Anticipating & early detection

28 Feb 2020 - 21 Mar 2020 Phase 2 Strategies to contain

22 Mar 2020 - 27 Apr 2020 Phase 3 Policies to control & mitigate

28 Apr 2020 - May 2021 Phase 4 Opening up and eradication

Figure 4.2: New Zealand timeline, 2020–2021.

Each of these levels indicate the public health and social measures to be taken, such as staying at home, severe travel restrictions, and school closures during Level 4.

As seen in Figure 4.2, once the Alert Levels were developed, almost immediately the country went into Level 4. In Horton's (2020, 72) words, when the Prime Minister 'called a national emergency on 25 March.... (H)er clear, consistent, and confident messaging to the public was a model of political choreography in a crisis.'

This lockdown was followed by a progressive lifting at the end of April 2020 when there were very few cases. This has led some to observe that '(t)he lockdown implemented in New Zealand was remarkable for its stringency and its brevity' (Robert, 2020, 569). In terms of economic policies, in Phase 2 a NZ$12.1 billion economic assistance package was secured, consisting of NZ$500 million towards health, NZ$8.7 towards businesses and jobs, NZ$2.8 billion to income support measures; this was followed by a NZ$50 billion recovery package announced in Phase 4 in the 2020 budget.[9] When turning to R&D funding this was found throughout the phases as follows: NZ$3 million towards COVID-19 research in Phase 2; NZ$3.8 million for projects and clinical trials in Phase 3; and NZ$6.75 million towards projects on detecting antibodies, developing a simple ventilator, and vaccine research in Phase 4.[10]

New Zealand interestingly shows how throughout the four phases in our typology there were very tight border/travel restrictions. This started right at the early phases in February (when there was a ban on travellers from mainland China) and March (when there were strict self-isolation measures for those entering and a later travel ban where all borders were closed to non-New Zealand residents), lasting well until Phase 4. This closing of international borders was done before most countries, and was based on the epidemiologists' advice (Mazey and Richardson, 2020, 564).

To indicate the success of this policy, Graph 4.4 plots the number of COVID cases (on a 7-day rolling average, y-left axis) and compares this with the number of people travelling in planes (measured in terms of seat capacity, y-right axis) between February 17 and December 28, 2020.

Graph 4.4 shows that as COVID-19 cases were starting to rise exponentially at the end of March and April 2020, there was a rapid fall in the number of international and domestic flights as borders closed. Seat capacity on planes would

---

9 On these see: https://www.beehive.govt.nz/release/121-billion-support-new-zealanders-and-business and https://www.treasury.govt.nz/information-and-services/new-zealand-economy/covid-19-economic-response/measures
10 For more information, see: https://covid19policywatch.org/policies/new-zealand

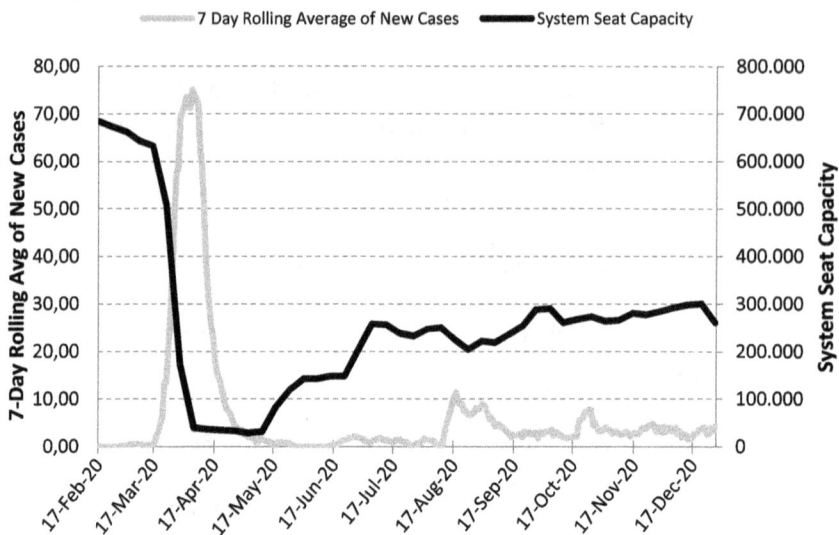

- - - - - 7 Day Rolling Average of New Cases   ▬▬▬System Seat Capacity

Graph 4.4: Flights and COVID-19 cases in New Zealand, February–December 2020. Source of data: CAPA Centre for Aviation and https://ourworldindata.org/

only start to rise well after the beginning of May, when there were virtually no new cases. Even as cases may have seen slight increases (i.e. local maxima) as the time series continues, the number of flights would concomitantly drop at those times. By January 2021 when traffic in New Zealand was around a third of what it as before the pandemic, only 10 % of flights were international.

We now turn our attention to Europe. In contrast to New Zealand, and like most of the world, countries such as Ireland and Germany experienced more than one wave. Examining both countries comparatively thus offers the opportunity to examine the 'feedback' mechanism of our model. By comparing the policies each state pursued after the first wave, we will demonstrate how some states successfully formulated necessary policies when reverting back to Phase 3 (policies to control and mitigate) when already in Phase 4 (opening up), while others did not.

Europe: comparing Ireland and Germany

Our comparative analysis of Ireland and Germany starts by examining the 7-day rolling average (on a normalized scale) of new confirmed COVID-19 cases over a

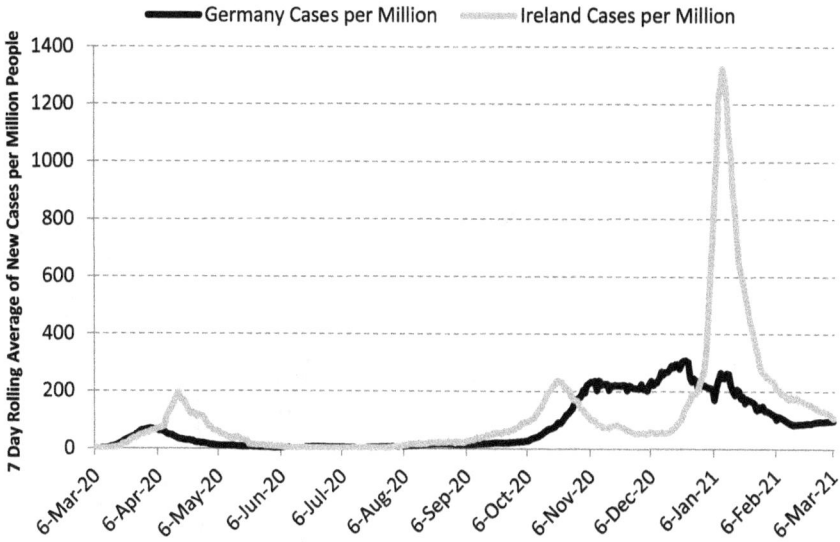

Graph 4.5: 7-Day rolling average of daily new confirmed cases per million people in Ireland and Germany, March 2020–March 2021. Source of data: https://ourworldindata.org/

one-year period, between March 6, 2020 and March 6, 2021. Graph 4.5 shows that Ireland experienced more waves than Germany and saw extremely high numbers of cases comparatively per capita.

This observation ostensibly leads one to the question: what policy differences were seen in the countries, particularly in the latter part of the series which saw a huge comparative spike in cases in Ireland around Christmas 2020? To answer this, Figure 4.3 considers the timeline of the first wave found in Ireland, from February to September 2020.[11]

Assessing the Irish performance against our typology, three positive points can be noted in the figure. First, in Phase 2 the country increased its healthcare spending by €435 million to tackle COVID-19. This is significant considering that the Irish health care system does not provide free universal coverage and is known for its accessibility problems for all patients where some of the best treat-

---

11 Beyond the main sources outlined in Appendix A and noted in this section, the following webpages have also been consulted in the development of our narrative and timelines for Ireland that may be useful for researchers investigating Ireland: https://www.gov.ie/en/ and https://data.oireachtas.ie/ For Germany, the following were also consulted: https://www.dw.com, https://www.deutschland.de, and https://www.euractiv.com/

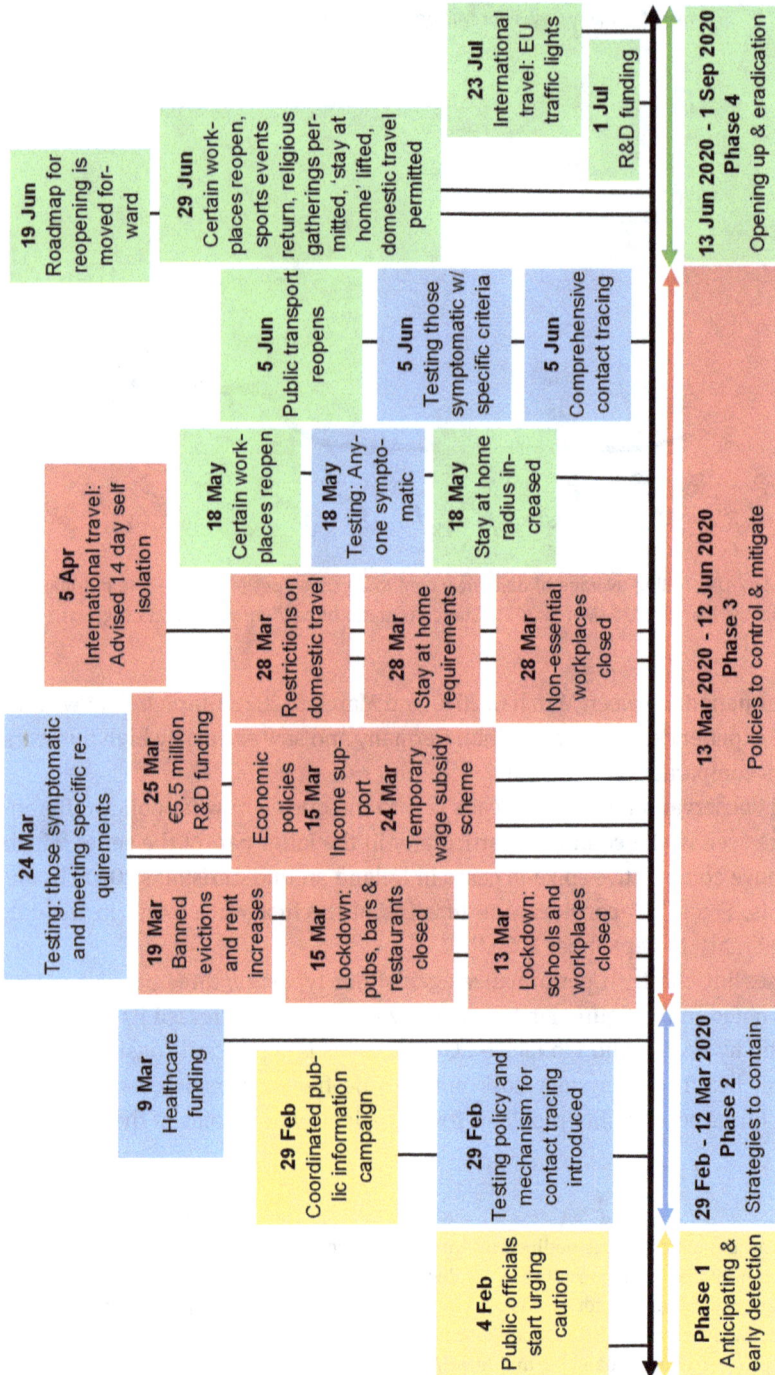

Figure 4.3: Key public policies in Ireland during Wave 1, February–September 2020.

ment comes from the private (not public) system.[12] Secondly, Phase 3 'lockdown' started on a gradual basis when the initial surge of cases took place before mid-March. This is in sharp contrast to its closest neighbour – the UK – which witnessed a delay in lockdown that started in late March.[13] In this regard, Prime Minister Leo Varadkar, who is a medical doctor by training, was praised for his quick and decisive action in taking concrete steps to control the virus early including pre-emptively cancelling St. Patrick's Day events while the virus was still contained.[14] Thirdly, Ireland formulated robust economic policies regarding both the pandemic unemployment payment of €203 per week for those out of work as a result of COVID-19, as well as a temporary wage subsidy scheme. Although R&D funding did not start in Phase 2, there were later rounds including of Science Foundation Ireland's funding worth €5.5 million.[15]

Nevertheless, Ireland's first wave saw policy developments were wanting on at least four fronts. The first shortcoming, in contrast to New Zealand, is that travel restrictions did not take place in the first two phases, and even in Phase 3 there was only advised isolation for international travellers and not a travel ban *per se*. Secondly, a comprehensive testing and contract tracing policy did not take place in the early part of the wave; in fact, the timeline illustrates how the definition for those who should be tested changed throughout the various phases. Third, there were some delays in starting a coordinated public information campaign that eventually manifested in Phase 2, even though there was some evidence that officials tried to urge some caution about the virus in Phase 1. Finally, the first wave itself saw no indication of any form of an initial (or even later) emergency action plan being produced in order to deal with the virus; instead, as we will see, this was only formulated at the start of the second wave.

Figure 4.4 considers policy developments in both the second and third waves that occurred between September 2020 and May 2021, which captures the feedback mechanism of our typology. It shows the main policies that were pursued during:

- Wave 2 – where Phase 3 started in early September 2020 as cases started to surge once again, while Phase 4 took place in the first two weeks of December 2020.

---

12 https://www.thejournal.ie/irish-healthcare-system-3242479-Feb2017/

13 See: https://www.bmj.com/content/370/bmj.m3166

14 See, for example, the *Globe and Mail*'s report on: https://www.theglobeandmail.com/world/article-leo-varadkar-lauded-for-steady-handling-of-covid-19-crisis-as-ireland/

15 https://www.sfi.ie/research-news/news/minister-harris-covid-19/

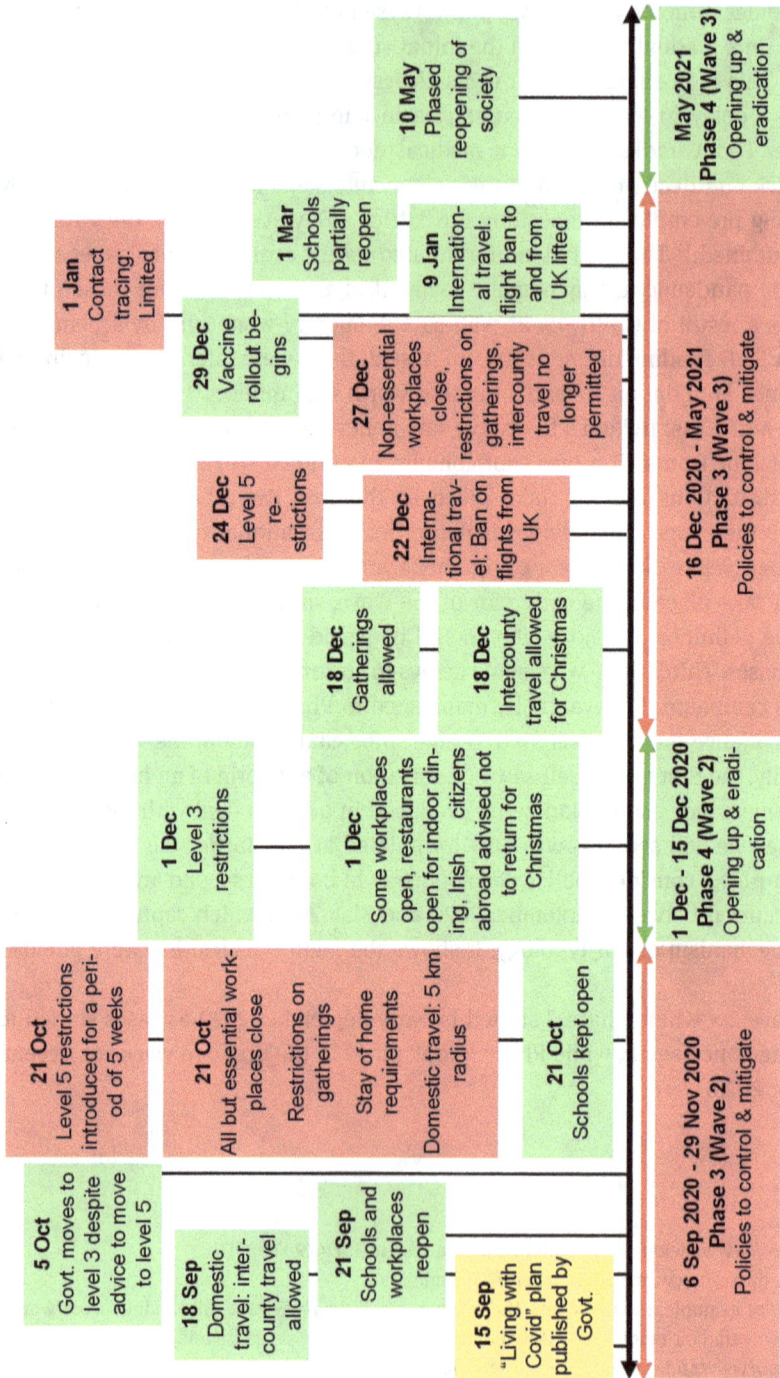

Figure 4.4: Key public policies in Ireland in Phases 3 and 4 of **Waves** 2 and 3.

- Wave 3 – Where Phase 3 started in mid-December when there was an initial surge again to mark the third wave, and whose 7-day average only started to dissipate and flatten in May 2021.

Figure 4.4 is illustrative of a marble cake: not only was a delayed emergency plan called 'Living with Covid' developed one wave late, but more importantly some opening up (green) policies were pursued during periods when the country should have been pursuing policies of control and mitigate (red), and vice versa. Key developments illustrating this are as follows:

- As cases initially surged in early September 2020, opening up policies on travel and schools took place. This, despite the National Public Health Emergency Team led by Dr. Tony Holohan urging in early October that full 'Level 5' lockdown should be implemented.[16] Nonetheless, Level 5 was only implemented by the government during the peak of Wave 2 at the end of October, almost seven weeks after the initial surge. Once Level 5 was announced, cases substantially dropped and some opening up policies took place in early December as the country entered Phase 4.
- By mid-December, however, an initial surge marked the start of the 3rd wave just as the alpha variant was causing an increase in cases in the UK.[17] Rather than adopt lockdown policies, the government allowed intercounty travel within Ireland and opened up gatherings for Christmas celebrations. The subsequent return to lockdown at the end of December came too late: the rise in cases had already gained momentum, resulting in Ireland's third wave being its largest both in terms of numbers and the sheer exponential growth experienced in such a short time (see Graph 4.5). The numbers were so high that by the beginning of the year the state did not have sufficient resources to be able to fully contact trace. Moreover, despite a ban on flights from the UK by December 22, given fears associated with the alpha variant, the government bizarrely eased travel restrictions and lifted the ban in early January, slightly before the peak of the 3rd wave.

In contrast to Ireland, Germany offers an example of a European state that pursued lockdown and opening up policies throughout waves as expected in Phases 3 and 4 of our typology respectively, offering a clear example of a (mostly) layer cake. To this end, Figure 4.5 considers developments during Phases 3 and 4 of

---

16 See: https://www.irishtimes.com/news/politics/timeline-nphet-level-5-recommendation-who-knew-what-and-when-1.4375677

17 See: https://www.thelancet.com/journals/lanres/article/PIIS2213-2600(21)00005-9/fulltext

the first wave in Germany between March and October 2020, and Phase 3 of the second wave that lasted between October 2020 and February 2021.

After the first COVID-19 cases were recorded at the end of February 2020, a surge occurred in early March at which time initial policies were pursued in specific regions where clusters had emerged, such as banning large events in Bavaria and North Rhine-Westphalia (Czypionka and Reiss, 2021, 299). Figure 4.5 captures that, while initial lockdown policies in Phase 3 were formulated at the state level, a coordinated approach was taken mid-March 2020. This approach was thus led by the federal government of Dr. Angela Merkel, where a series of restrictions were announced, including closing non-essential shops, businesses, schools and sports facilities (Czypionka and Reiss, 2021, 298). Reflective of the country's relatively tough stance on international movements, there were also border closures with Austria, Denmark, France, Luxembourg and Switzerland as well as restricted air travel with other EU and non-EU countries. March also witnessed a major economic relief package of €156 billion to deal with the pandemic, which was supplemented with a €130 billion aid package in late June. As the month of March progressed there was tightening of lockdown, with stay at home orders, closure of restaurants and limiting public gatherings to two people that are socially distanced (the 'Contact Ban').[18]

While these early actions have been described as exemplary,[19] there is evidence of some conflict between levels of governance where federal officials in the 'Corona Cabinet' sometimes saw 'conflictual telephone conferences with state governors' (Czypionka and Reiss, 2021, 306). Perhaps because of this, the gradual relaxing of lockdown that took place from mid-April even though the country still found itself in Phase 3 was led by individual Länder (states). This resulted in non-coordinated action between May and June (Czypionka and Reiss, 2021, 311), reflected in the one 'green' policy box in Phase 3 of Wave 1 in Figure 4.5. Opening up policies continued when expected as per our typology throughout Phase 4 of Wave 1 during June and October 2020, including opening up flights and the pioneering test of staging a concert in Leipzig in August 2020 with pre- and post-event detection tests to better understand how to control the virus' spread in large events.[20]

What is of relevance to our comparative analysis with Ireland is how Germany's Phase 3 of Wave 2 (between October 2020 and February 2021) contrasts with

---

18 On the 'Contact Ban' of March 22, see: https://edition.cnn.com/world/live-news/coronavirus-outbreak-03-22-20/h_7c002a4c0abcb50250580f6e376f1b9d
19 https://ourworldindata.org/covid-exemplar-germany-2020?country=
20 See: https://www.npr.org/sections/coronavirus-live-updates/2020/08/24/905554790/german-experiment-tests-how-coronavirus-spreads-at-a-concert?t=1621591361319

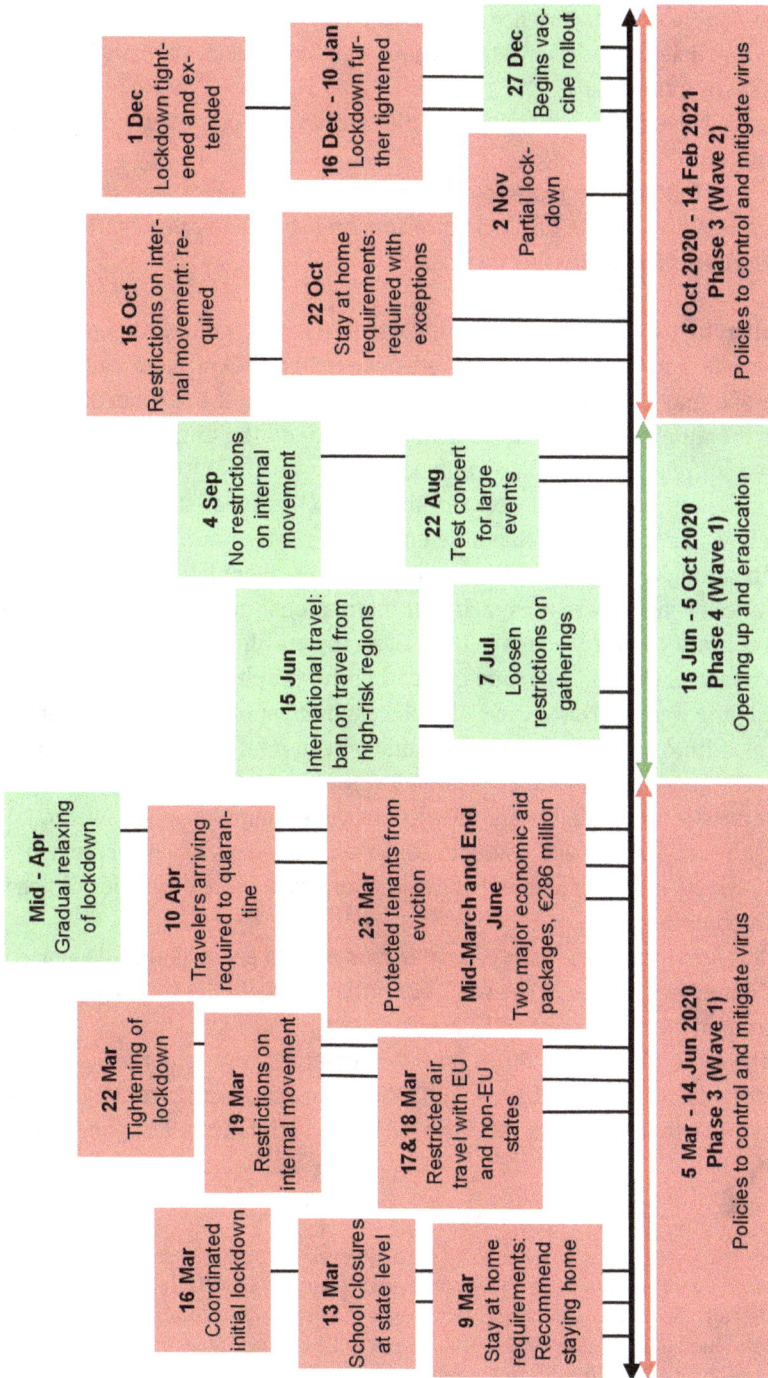

Figure 4.5: Key policies in Germany in Phases 3 and 4 of Wave 1 and Phase 3 of Wave 2.

the Irish marble cake experience discussed above. Germany maintained stricter lockdown policies than Ireland throughout the time period, particularly during Christmas. In more detail:

- in early November a one-month partial lockdown (lockdown light) was announced;
- this was followed by more restrictions in early December, and, finally,
- there was an effective full lockdown from mid-December until early January 2021 given increasing case numbers.[21]

Comparing the two countries shows that while Ireland encouraged people to actively reunite and enjoy holidays together, Germany took a more cautious approach: one may reasonably argue that this did not result in an uncontrollable spike in the number of cases in Germany during and after Christmas, as was experienced in Ireland as seen in Graph 4.5.

To close our comparison between the two EU member states and as mentioned above, another policy that differentiates the two countries is travel restrictions. Accordingly, Graphs 4.6 and 4.7 consider the evolution of the number of COVID-19 cases against seat capacity on international and domestic flights between February 10 and December 28 in Germany and Ireland respectively.

Six observations can be made comparing the Graphs 4.6 and 4.7:

- While the week of March 2 saw the highest number of flights in 2020 for Germany with 4,854,293 million seats, this occurred later in Ireland where the highest number was found in March 9 with 747,893 seats. This demonstrates that a reduction in flights and restrictions were comparatively slower to take place in Ireland. We will use both of these numbers as our measurement of 'pre-COVID' numbers before flight restrictions took place during lockdown in both countries.
- In the first lockdown, both countries managed to see a similar decrease in the number of flights: in the week of April 20, 2020, both saw a seat capacity of around 7% from pre-COVID levels.
- In the week of April 25, 2020, however, Ireland saw a remarkable spike in flights, rising to 62% of pre-COVID flight capacity, which contrasts to the 17% in Germany. This is reflective of Ireland's relatively lax policy at the

---

21 On the first partial lockdown for a month starting November 2020 see: https://www.dw.com/en/coronavirus-germany-to-impose-one-month-partial-lockdown/a-55421241. On the second starting in early December, see: https://www.theguardian.com/world/2020/nov/25/germany-to-decide-next-round-of-covid-restrictions. And on the full lockdown from December 2020 see: https://www.bbc.com/news/world-europe-55292614.

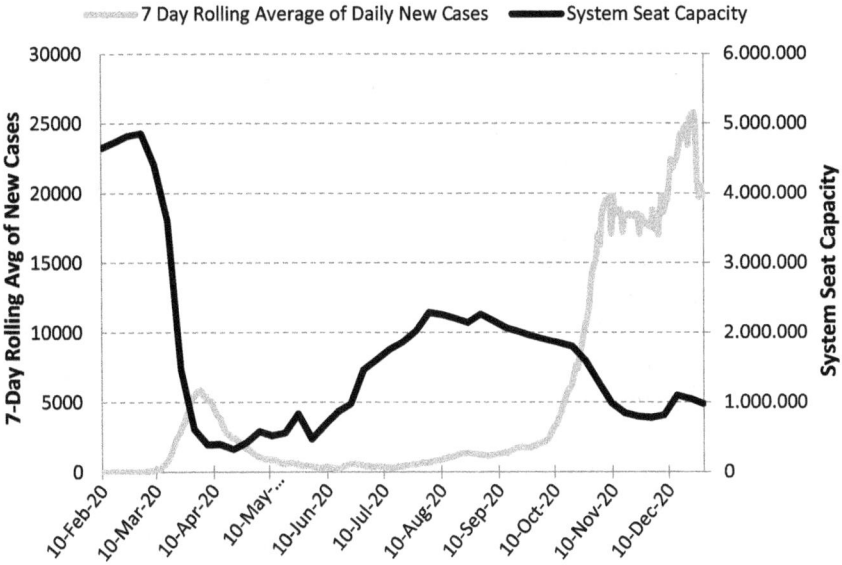

Graph 4.6: Flights and COVID-19 cases in Germany, February–December 2020. Source of data: CAPA Centre for Aviation and https://ourworldindata.org/

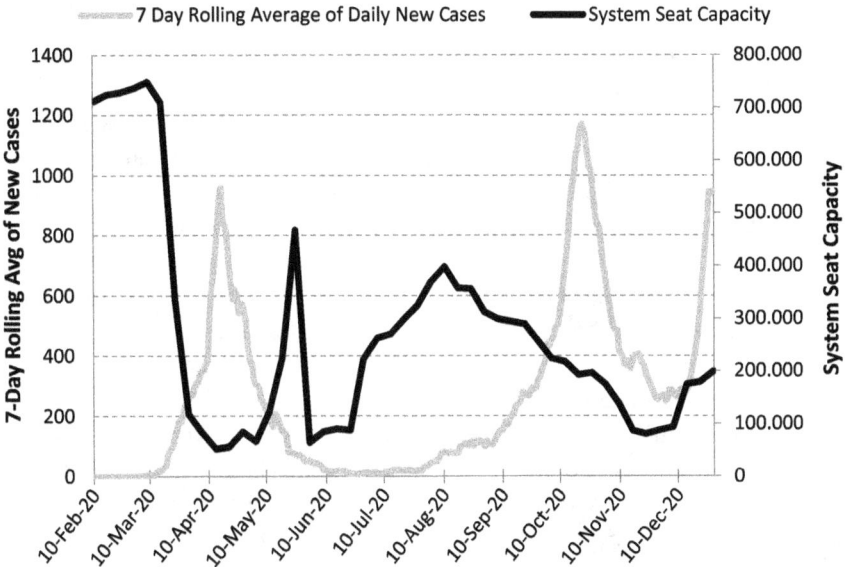

Graph 4.7: Flights and COVID-19 cases in Ireland, February–December 2020. Source of data: CAPA Centre for Aviation and https://ourworldindata.org/

time of only advising new entrants to self-isolate without having a firm policy on travel restrictions/bans at the time.

- Over the summer, similar curves are seen in both. But while Germany never attained more than 50% of pre-COVID numbers at any time, Ireland saw 53% in the week of August 10.
- Interestingly during the week of December 7, 2020, Ireland had 12.5% of pre-COVID seat capacity, while Germany had around 17%. This helps demonstrates the strong impact of Ireland's full (Level 5) lockdown at the time when compared to Germany's partial lockdown.
- Nevertheless, once Ireland opened up for Christmas, flight numbers by the week of December 28 would rise to around 27% of pre-Covid capacity, compared to 20% in Germany.

Crossing the Atlantic sees a similar story of states that had stark differences in COVID-19 cases and experienced different policy choices, even more than Ireland and Germany. The next section thus turns to the experience of both Canada and the US.

Canada and the US: very different neighbours

By early June 2021, the US had experienced close to 600,000 deaths due to COVID-19, while Canada saw over 25,500. On a normalized scale measuring the number of deaths per capita, this same data in the US translates into 181 deaths/100K population, which is close to three times that of Canada at 68/ 100K.[22] These huge differences are also captured in Graph 4.8 that considers the evolution of the daily new confirmed cases per 100 million people between the start of the pandemic in March 6, 2020 until June 2, 2021.

Graph 4.8 shows that case numbers from the US were consistently higher than its northern neighbour until early April 2021. Interestingly, from April 9, this trend is reversed when the lines intersect. This can be best understood as a function of vaccinations: on this date the percentage of the population in the US receiving the first dose of the vaccine was over 34%, while those having received two doses was over 20%. In comparison, at that time in Canada only 18% had received the first dose, while the percentage of those receiving a second dose was a paltry 2%.[23]

---

22 Data taken on June 2, 2021, from https://coronavirus.jhu.edu/data/mortality
23 Based on data found in https://ourworldindata.org/

USA 7 Day Rolling Average per Million People
Canada 7 Day Rolling Average per Million People

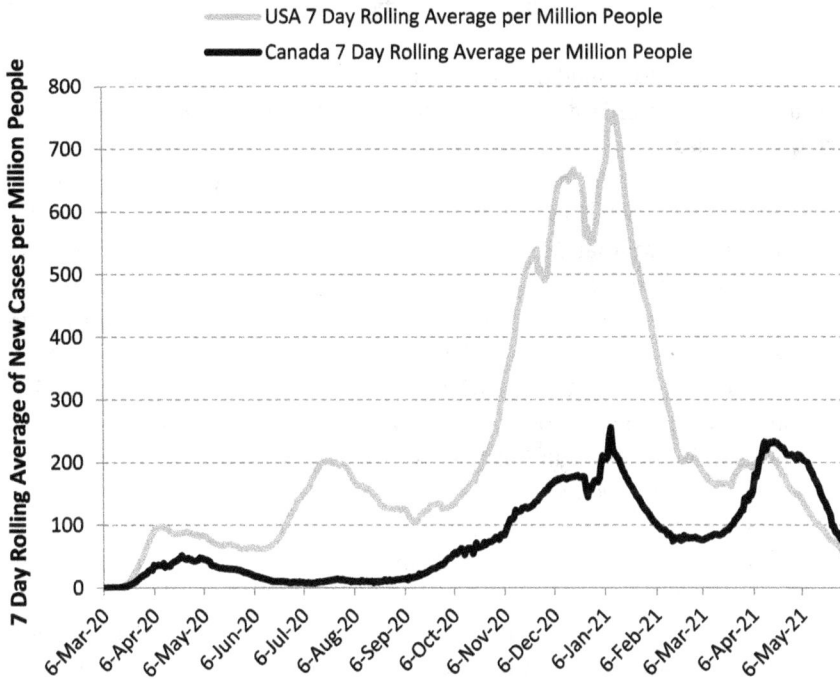

Graph 4.8: Daily confirmed COVID-19 cases per million people in the US and Canada, March 2020–June 2021. Source of data: https://ourworldindata.org/

The differences in the numbers shown in Graph 4.8 reflect the policies (or, lack thereof) adopted throughout the pandemic by both countries before there was a vaccine solution, and in this section we consider policy dynamics in the first wave of the virus.

Comparison between the two countries is significant not only because of the divergent numbers of cases and deaths between these geographically close neighbours, but also because both are federal systems.

In the case of the US, Singer et al. (2021, 478–9) note that while 'health care in the United States sits at the nexus of federal and state control, with states overseeing many policy choices and implementation... in times of crisis, the United States public health system depends on the federal government to coordinate policy and distribute resources and expertise to the states.' During COVID-19, however, this did not happen. This is because under President Trump's leadership (better said, absence of leadership), individual states were burdened with the responsibility to contain, control and mitigate the virus without much federal guidance or resources. This resulted in 'widely heterogenous responses across the United States' during Trump's term in office (Singer et al., 2020, 479; see also Kettl, 2020).

When turning to Canada, during times of non-crisis, health policy can be seen as tending towards decentralization: while the federal government plays a key role in health policy, 'provincial and territorial (PT) governments are responsible for most public health measures and the delivery of health services' (Fafard et al., 2021, 461). However, when it comes to emergencies more generally, experience has shown that Canada rallies around the central government to offer leadership. As Migone (2020b, 392) argues, Canadian history demonstrates the importance of 'crisis federalism' when there was a return to centralization '... during a period of emergency or stress.' Thus, in contrast to the US experience, it comes as no surprise that Canada witnessed a 'wave of unprecedented interjurisdictional cooperation' to confront COVID-19 under the federal leadership of Prime Minister Justin Trudeau (Migone, 2020b, 397). Although the Canadian experience was far from perfect given some provincial differences as we will see, the relatively unified response when compared to the US not only gained citizen approval, but also international comparisons that the countries were like 'night and day' during the first wave.[24]

It is thus relatively easy to draw a timeline for the Canadian federal government response during the first wave of COVID-19 precisely because there was more of a coordinated, unified approach to deal with the pandemic when compared to the US, which effectively allowed individual states to 'go it alone'. Figure 4.6 shows this timeline, which demonstrates that the country pursued policies that were largely expected of it in the different phases of our typology.[25]

The Canadian timeline is generally representative of a 'layer cake', although more 'marble' is seen when compared to New Zealand. Noteworthy initiatives at the beginning of the pandemic before cases surged included $500 million for critical health system needs, which was effectively a transfer to provincial governments that anticipated their need to deal with COVID, and $275 million towards vaccine and antiviral research while in Phase 2. Nevertheless, it falls short in some ways; for example, in Phase 1 there was neither an initial emergency action plan developed by the federal government, nor the start of a coordinated information campaign. Further, while the country saw a unified lockdown policy as cases surged in March 2020 (discussed below), during the end of

---

24 See: https://www.theguardian.com/world/2020/jul/09/canada-coronavirus-us-justin-trudeau-donald-trump

25 Beyond the main sources outlined in Appendix A and noted in this section, the following webpages have also been consulted in the development of our narrative and timeline for Canada: https://www.canada.ca/en.html, https://www.parl.ca/ and https://pm.gc.ca/en

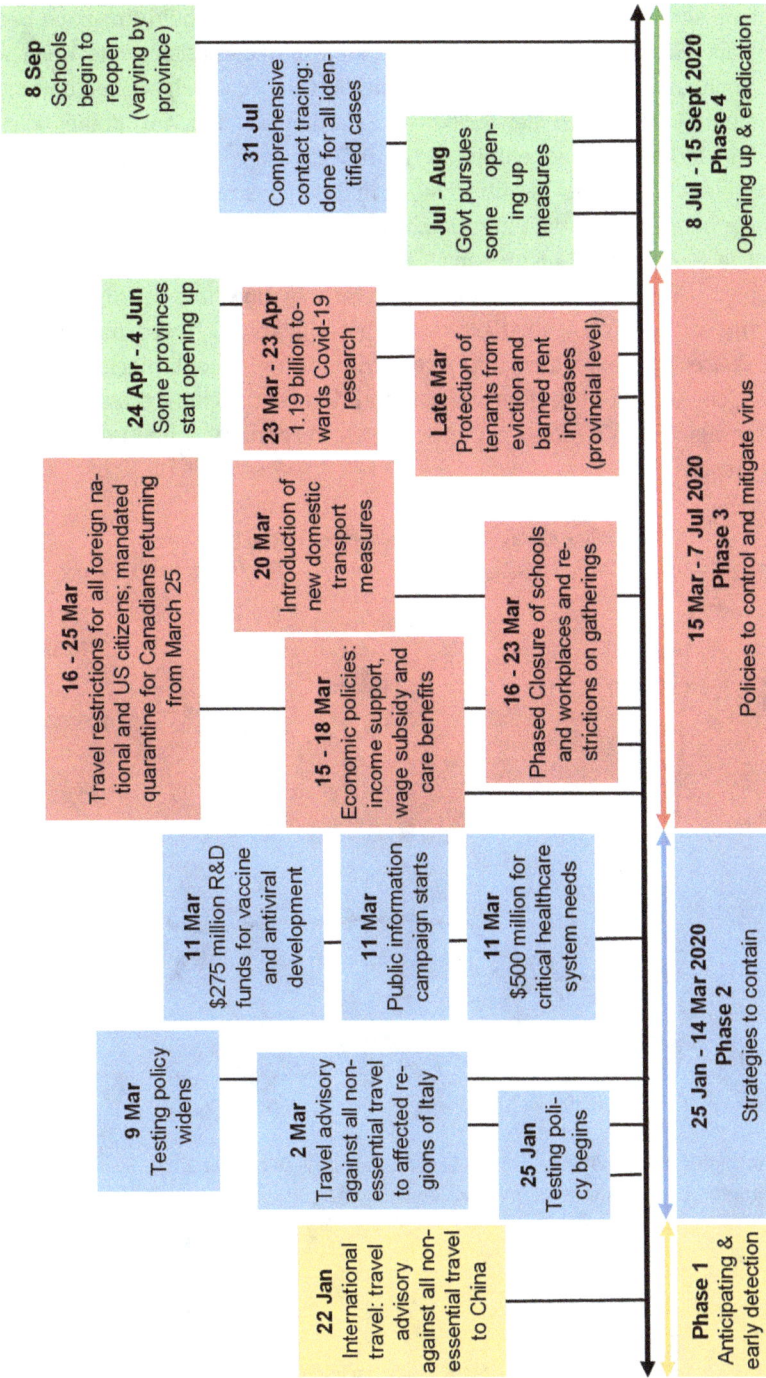

Figure 4.6: Canada timeline, Wave 1, January–September 2020.

Phase 3 we see some 'green' policies when the country should not have been opening up. This points to the idea that some provinces started to open up early in some aspects, as seen in the province of Québec which opened daycares and elementary schools in May 2020.[26] As Fafard et al. (2021, 461) argue, 'variation in the start date of reopening did not reflect case count nor risk.'

There are at least four key dimensions that demonstrate the similarities and differences between Canadian and US policy choices (or absence of). The first dimension relates to travel restrictions. Compared to other states we have examined such as New Zealand, Canada was relatively slow to stop flights: while the country did advise against travel in Phases 1 and 2, it was not until the start of Phase 3 in mid-March that a reduction of flights took place. Graph 4.9 plots seat capacity of both international and domestic flights against the 7-day rolling average of COVID cases in Canada between February 17 and December 28, 2020, inclusive.

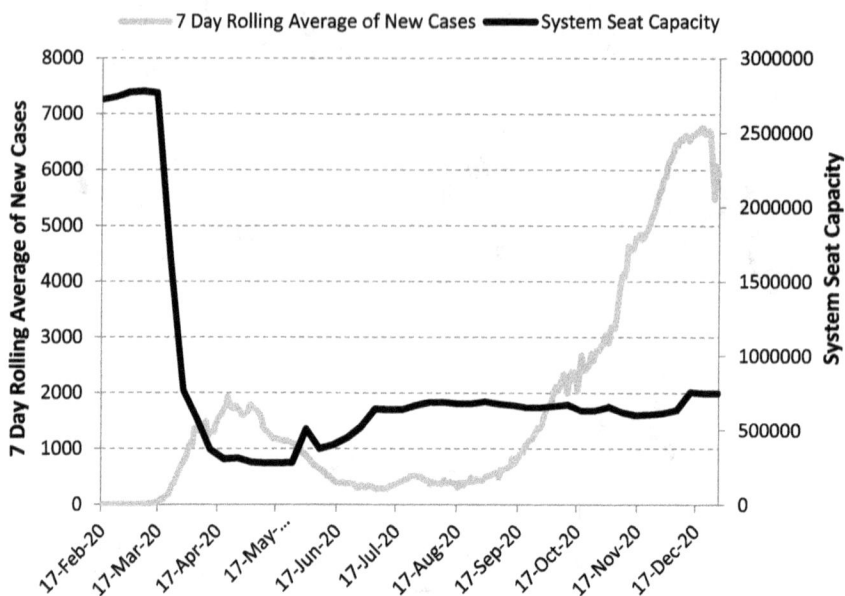

Graph 4.9: Flights and COVID-19 Cases in Canada, February–December 2020. Source of data: CAPA Centre for Aviation and https://ourworldindata.org/

---

26 See: https://globalnews.ca/news/6928407/quebec-schools-daycares-reopen-coronavirus/

It shows that seat capacity for March 16 was the highest for the time series (with 2.77 million seats, which we will use as a figure for 'Pre-COVID' flight capacity). After mid-March, the number of flights dramatically declined, reaching a nadir of around 10% of pre-COVID levels by May 25. While this number would gradually increase to a local maximum of around 25% of pre-COVID levels in the week of August 30 due to summer travel, it remained mostly around this level as case numbers rose in the latter half of 2020. This relatively prudent approach can be explained based on a clear opening up policy with 'Canada's flight plan' for safe air travel that was launched in mid-August 2020.[27]

In contrast, the friendly skies over the US remained comparatively open, where the number of flights remained high as the number of cases were surging. Even when flights were reduced at their lowest point in May, comparative figures of both international and domestic flights see that the US operated at over 20% of its pre-COVID flight capacity (compared to Canada's 10%, as discussed above), over 50% during August (compared to Canada's 25%), and close to 60% at Christmas (compared to slightly more than 25% in Canada).

One may reasonably question: how could this be the case if early in the pandemic the US imposed a travel ban from EU states in early March, and had mutually agreed some days later to close borders with Canada and Mexico over several months? The answer is based on the fact that around 80% of all pre-COVID airline seats in the US are on domestic routes and were untouched by these international restrictions.[28] Graph 4.10 considers domestic and international seat capacity separately in the US between February 17 and December 28, 2020, as well as the 7-day rolling average of cases in the country.

This graph demonstrates that international flights had decreased at one point in early May to 7.5% of pre-COVID capacity, and then slightly increased over time. In contrast, domestic flights went from their lowest point in May of around 25% of pre-COVID levels, and then surged to levels of over 50% capacity in August. This then jumped to 60% by Thanksgiving in November and Christmas at the end of December when domestic travel was at its highest.

A second dimension that differentiates the two countries relates to testing. The Canadian timeline shows that testing policy started and extended in

---

27 For more details on Transport Minister Garneau's plan, please see the press release of August 14, 2020 at: https://www.canada.ca/en/transport-canada/news/2020/08/government-of-canada-releases-canadas-flight-plan-for-safe-air-travel.html

28 In comparison, Canada's Pre-COVID seat capacity in March 2020 was as follows: international seats constituted 60% of all seats, and domestic 40%. As such, international restrictions on flights would have a stronger impact in Canada, particular as many of these flights are between the US and Canada (whose border was closed for months).

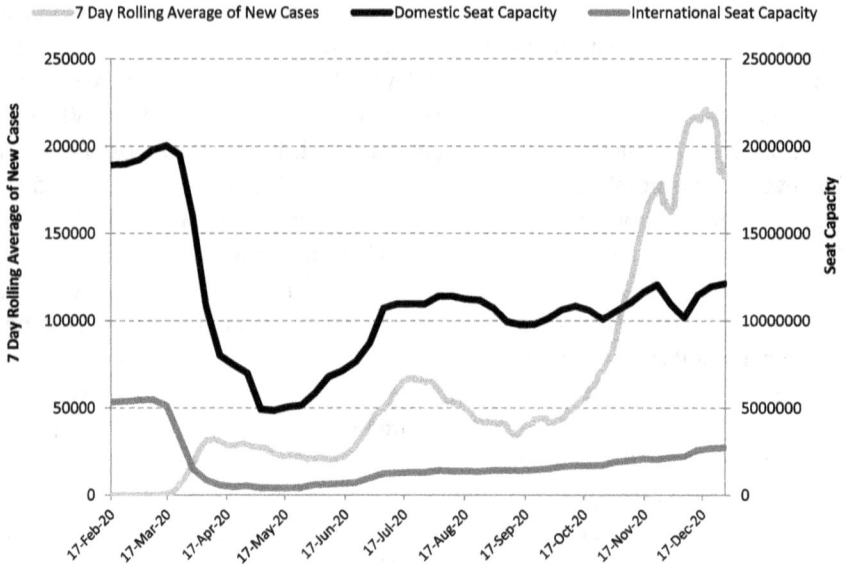

Graph 4.10: International and domestic flights and COVID-19 cases in the US. Source of data: CAPA Centre for Aviation and https://ourworldindata.org/

Phase 2, albeit with some early glitches in jurisdictions such as Ontario and Québec given a limited supply of diagnostic tests (Fafard et al., 2021). A comprehensive contact tracing policy, however, was only established some months later in July, when the country had seen reduced case numbers as seen in the blue box over Phase 4.

Even though Canada's performance on this second dimension was not optimal, it was still more robust than the US. While the public health agency, the CDC (the Centers for Disease Control), pursued screenings on those entering major US cities in February 2020, testing policy was wanting on many grounds as the first cases were emerging. This is reflected in an example from Singer et al. (2021, 480) that demonstrates the lack of unified response:

> Two individuals in California died in early February, but it was more than two months before their deaths were attributed to COVID-19... because they did not meet the criteria for testing, which was still required to be completed at the CDC in Atlanta.... Even as the federal government began decentralizing testing to the states, it was mired in a faulty rollout that did not standardize testing procedures or access to testing supplies. Thus, testing kits were

not distributed equally, regardless of population size, and localities encountered many delays as a result of contaminated testing materials.

On a third dimension, Canada experienced a more unified response to lockdown, with: a phased closure of schools, workplaces and restrictions on gatherings; clear protocols for those taking a domestic flight or train ride (such as having to take a pre-boarding health check); and quarantine for international arrivals. In contrast, the US's third phase (between mid-March and the end of May) of its first wave was characterized by disunity where the initiative to pursue lockdown measures was largely left to individual states and/or organizations themselves. As Singer et al. (2021, 481) explain, 'the failures of the Trump administration to respond to the virus became apparent with schools and universities, professional sports leagues, and many other organizations shutting down of their own accord or in response to subnational regulations.'

Finally, both countries pursued economic policies to deal with the negative impact of lockdown. In Canada, this included the Canada Emergency Response Benefit (CERB), the Canada Emergency Wage Subsidy, and income support to households. The country also saw two major R&D packages of $192 million and $1 billion announced in March and April respectively. The US similarly earmarked funds most notably through the CARES Act (Coronavirus Aid, Relief, and Economic Security Act) of late March 2020. This included billions towards, amongst other concepts, direct cash payments to individuals and households, unemployment benefits, and relief to businesses.[29] One shortcoming of the economic relief offered was that the federal government failed to offer the necessary financial support to the states. This meant that while 'federal government handed off authority to states to combat COVID-19, the financial burden was also taken up by subnational governments,' which subsequently incurred large debts (Singer et al., 2021, 484).

We now turn to compare public policies formulated by India, South Africa and Chile.

India, South Africa, and Chile: the large waves

This section comparatively examines these three countries for two main reasons. First, as seen earlier in Graph 4.2, the cumulative deaths in the first part of the pandemic in 2020 increased exponentially in all three countries. Second, as seen

---

29 For more details on the CARES Act, see Singer et al., 2021, 482–4

below, all three experienced first waves of generally longer duration than other states previously examined, with a longer time period for when Phase 3 policies to control and mitigate the virus should have been pursued. For example, in the case of India the first wave lasted over a year, where Phase 2 of our typology started at the end of January 2020, Phase 3 at the end of March 2020, and Phase 4 did not start until early February 2021.

While our examination will compare developments in the first wave of all three states, it is significant to note that all three experienced very large second waves that were bigger than the first. This is not dissimilar to other countries previously examined. Yet, the magnitude of the second wave in some of the countries in this section was simply astonishing. This was particularly seen in India which at one point experienced hundreds of thousands of new daily cases in April 2021 when it was ravaged with the Indian (delta) variant of the virus. This resulted in India's second wave having a peak almost four times larger than the first as seen in Graph 4.11.

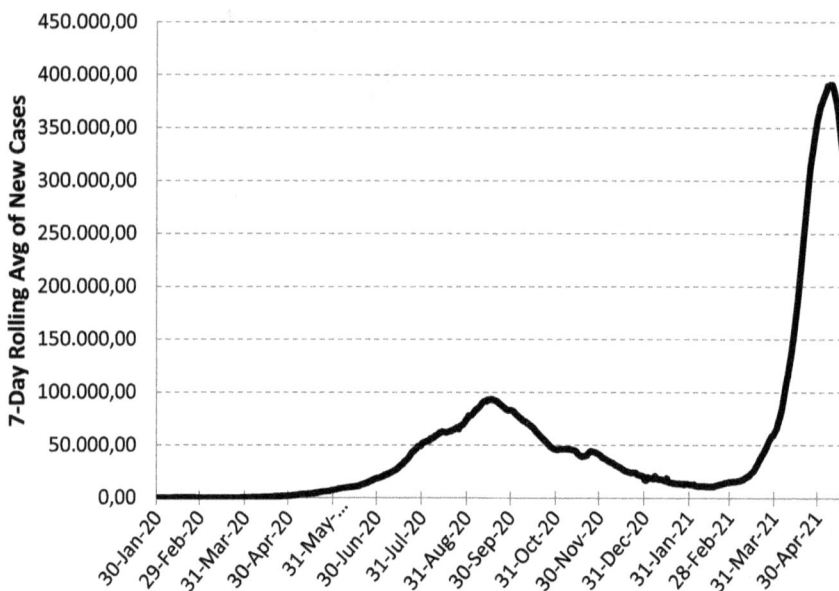

Graph 4.11: India 7-day rolling average of cases, January 2020–May 2021. Source of data: https://ourworldindata.org/

To capture the public policy developments in the first wave of all three states, Figure 4.7 considers India; Figure 4.8, South Africa; and Figure 4.9, Chile.[30]

Comparing the actions of all three in the early part of the timeline shows that, in contrast to most of the states previously discussed, there were early attempts to develop an initial emergency action plan. While in South Africa this took place in Phase 2, in India and Chile an attempt was made right in Phase 1 itself. Other similarities in the countries' timelines include that all three later pursued major economic stimulus measures to deal with COVID-19, including RS 20 lakh crore ($308 billion) in the case of India, an extraordinary budget of R500 billion in South Africa, and $11.75 billion in Chile.[31]

More significantly, as the timelines continue, the 'marble cake' seen in all three is fascinatingly similar but slightly different to other states seen before: these three countries started lockdown too quickly while in Phase 2 of our typology, only to then open up too early in Phase 3 when case numbers were still surging.

In more detail, on a first dimension, some lockdown policies (in red boxes) were pursued early during Phase 2 (indicated by the blue zone at the bottom of the black arrows of the timelines). In all three countries this included, for example, closing schools and restricting gatherings in mid-March, before a surge in cases occurred. This indicates that all three were proactive in pursuing lockdown early.

On a second dimension, all three countries were proactive in lifting lockdown early, pursuing opening up policies (green boxes) when still in the Phase 3 red zone. This was seen as follows:

- *India:* starting in March, India witnessed one of the longest lockdown periods in the world: 68 days. Although some have argued that this was a cen-

---

30 Beyond the main sources outlined in Appendix A and noted in this section, the following webpages have also been consulted in the development of our narrative and timelines for: India, https://www.mohfw.gov.in/ and https://pib.gov.in/; for South Africa, https://www.gov.za/ and https://sacoronavirus.co.za/ ; and for Chile, https://www.gob.cl/, https://www.minsal.cl/

31 Particularly impressive was the Rs 20 lakh crore ($308 billion) stimulus package by the Indian government, where more information can be seen here: https://economictimes.indiatimes.com/news/economy/finance/latest-stimulus-package-among-largest-in-the-world/articleshow/75701976.cms. Similarly, South marked R500 million in its extraordinary budget: https://mg.co.za/article/2020-04-21-ramaphosa-announces-r500-billion-covid-19-package-for-south-africa/.

And Chile announced a major stimulus plan equivalent to $11.75 billion, whose details can be seen at: https://www.bloomberg.com/news/articles/2020-03-19/chile-s-government-announces-11-75-billion-stimulus-plan

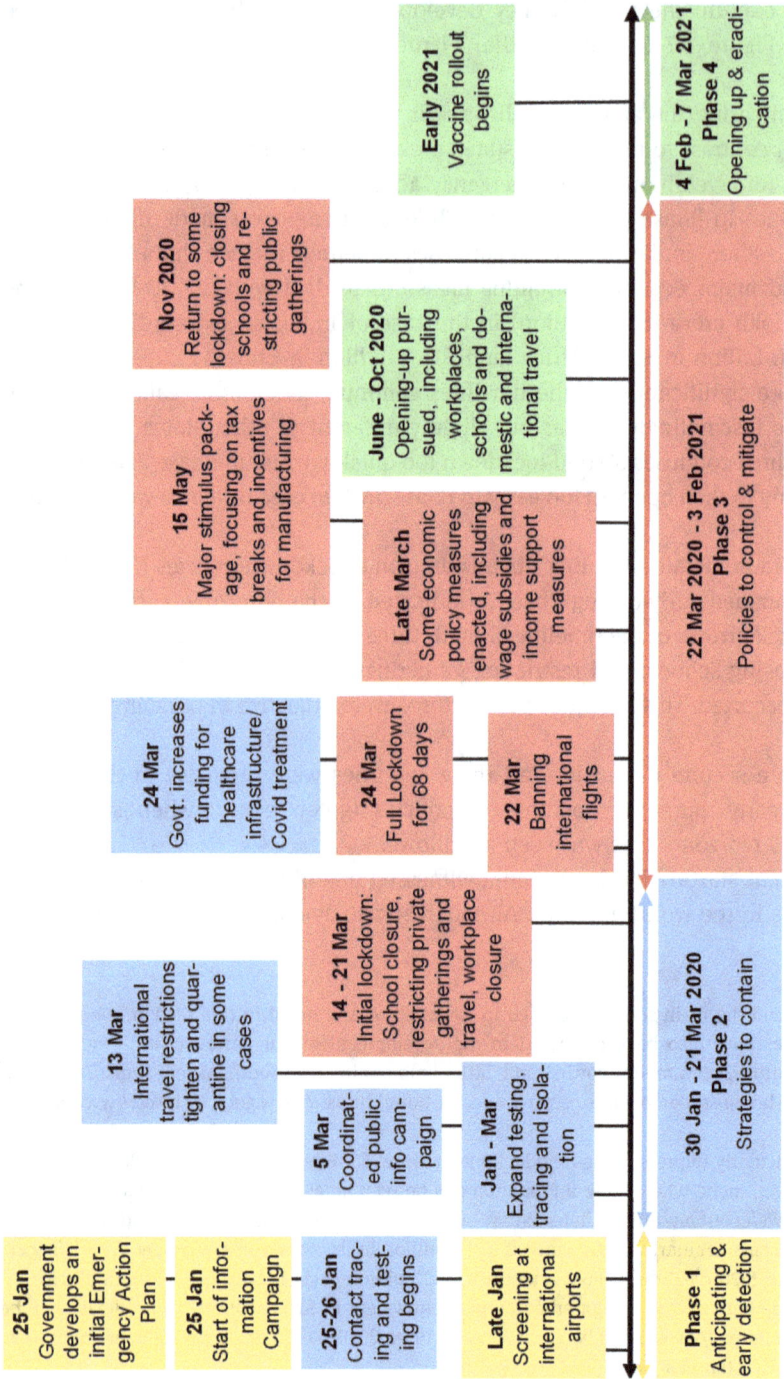

Figure 4.7: India timeline, Wave 1, January 2020–March 2021.

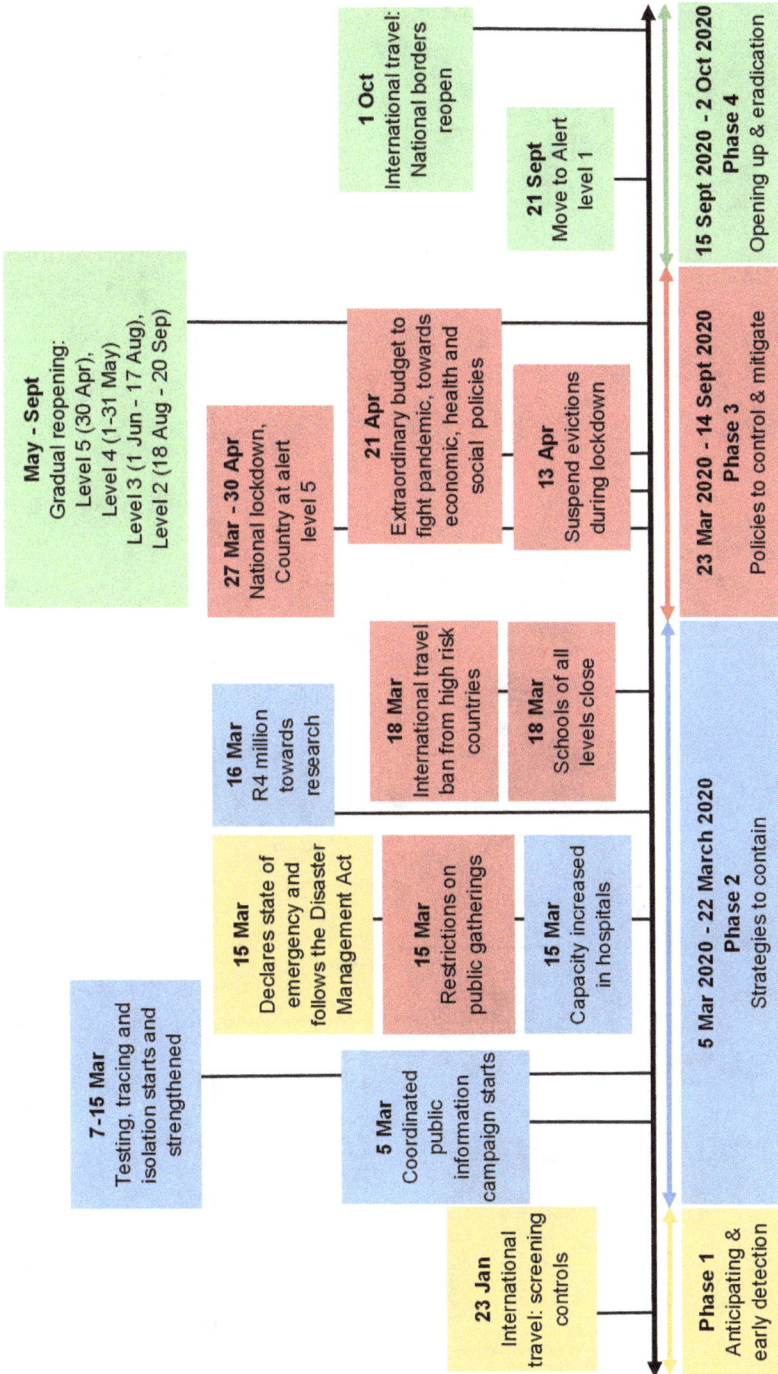

23 Jan International travel: screening controls

Phase 1 Anticipating & early detection

5 Mar Coordinated public information campaign starts

7-15 Mar Testing, tracing and isolation starts and strengthened

15 Mar Declares state of emergency and follows the Disaster Management Act

15 Mar Restrictions on public gatherings

15 Mar Capacity increased in hospitals

5 Mar 2020 - 22 March 2020 Phase 2 Strategies to contain

16 Mar R4 million towards research

18 Mar International travel ban from high risk countries

18 Mar Schools of all levels close

27 Mar – 30 Apr National lockdown, Country at alert level 5

21 Apr Extraordinary budget to fight pandemic, towards economic, health and social policies

13 Apr Suspend evictions during lockdown

23 Mar 2020 - 14 Sept 2020 Phase 3 Policies to control & mitigate

May - Sept Gradual reopening: Level 5 (30 Apr). Level 4 (1-31 May) Level3 (1 Jun - 17 Aug), Level 2 (18 Aug - 20 Sep)

21 Sept Move to Alert level 1

1 Oct International travel: National borders reopen

15 Sept 2020 - 2 Oct 2020 Phase 4 Opening up & eradication

Figure 4.8: South Africa timeline, Wave 1, March–October 2020.

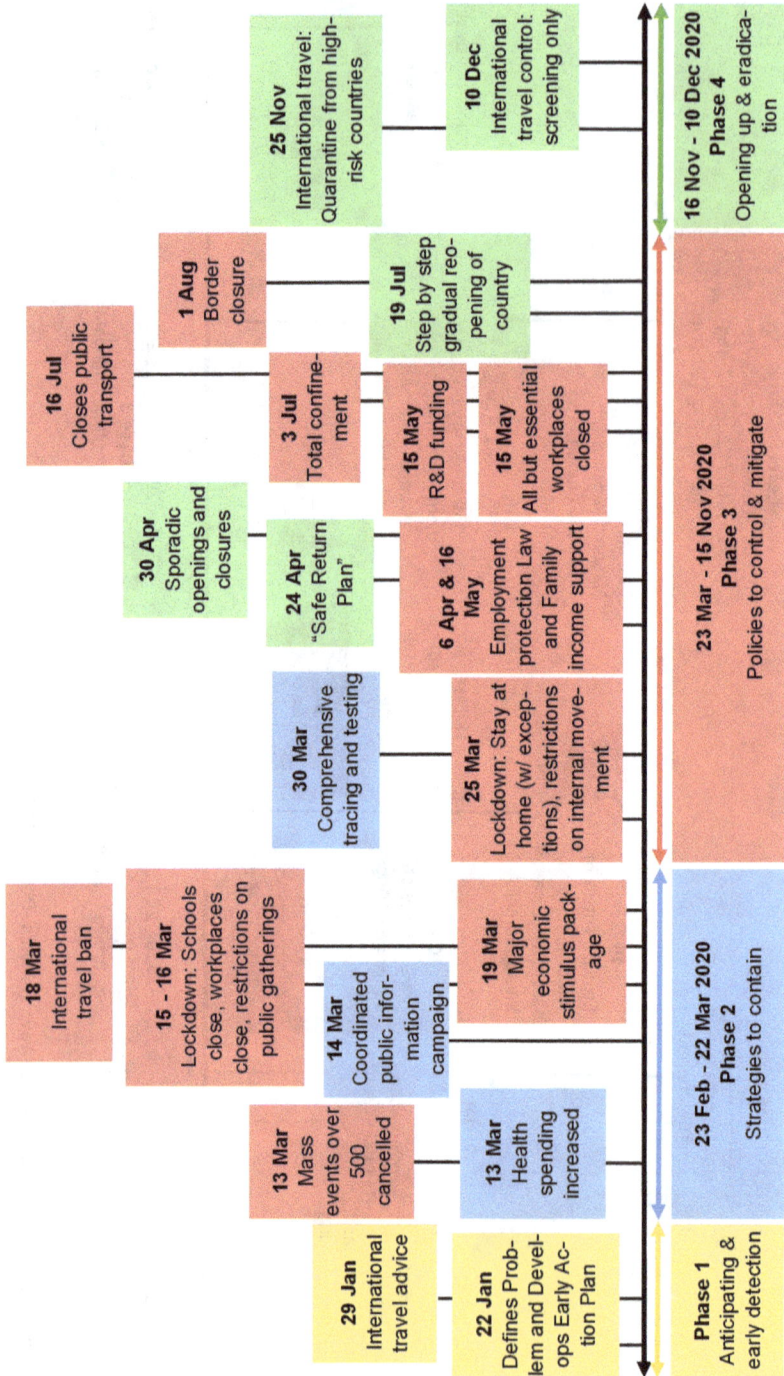

Figure 4.9: Chile timeline, Wave 1, February–December 2020.

tralized, authoritarian decision unilaterally taken by Prime Minister Nodi's government without consultation with experts (Raj, 2021, 180), others such as the WHO praised the lockdown as being 'tough and timely' (Horton, 2020, 73).[32] Regardless of how the lockdown can be characterized, opening up took place with regard to workplaces, schools and travel during June and October 2020. This opening occurred during a time period when cases were mostly on the rise (see Graph 4.8) and the country was still deep in Phase 3 of our typology.

- *South Africa:* The initial one month lockdown starting at the end of March was praised as being 'informed by scientific evidence' (Harris, 2020, 580). For testing, the government relied on the 'laboratory infrastructure that it used to monitor HIV and TB' (Harris, 2020, 585). Gradual reopening took place starting in May 2020, when the country moved from Level 4 to Level 2 on a phased basis until September. This early opening was a response to growing pressure to 'reopen and address the hunger and devastation the novel coronavirus and resulting lockdown had wrought', even though the WHO had advised against it (Harris, 2020, 585). As Graph 4.12 shows, the relaxing of Level 5 in early May came at a time when cases were rising, which would last until around the third week of July. Cases eventually flattened by late September/early October 2020.

- *Chile:* Its lockdown of late March 2020 was followed by a series of sporadic openings and closures at the end of April, including the opening of shopping centers as well as the reopening of schools that was eventually reversed given pressures by teachers, parents and students (Méndez, 2020, 527). As Méndez argues, the indecisiveness of the government during lockdown and the failure of their overall control and mitigation policies during Phase 3 is reflected in the fact that by June 2020 its '... erratic health measures placed Chile as one of the countries with the highest numbers of daily coronavirus cases relative to population size' (Méndez, 2020, 527). This eventually resulted in the resignation of the Health Minister Jaime Mañalich, heavily criticized for encouraging 'people to go back to normal, all while the curve was soaring upwards.'[33]

More research would need to be done to confirm this, but given the length of the waves of these three countries compared to other states, it may be reasonable to

---

32 For a good report on the lack of consultation, see also the BBC report at: https://www.bbc.com/news/world-asia-india-56561095
33 https://www.theguardian.com/global-development/2020/jun/14/chiles-health-minister-quits-over-government-response-to-covid-19

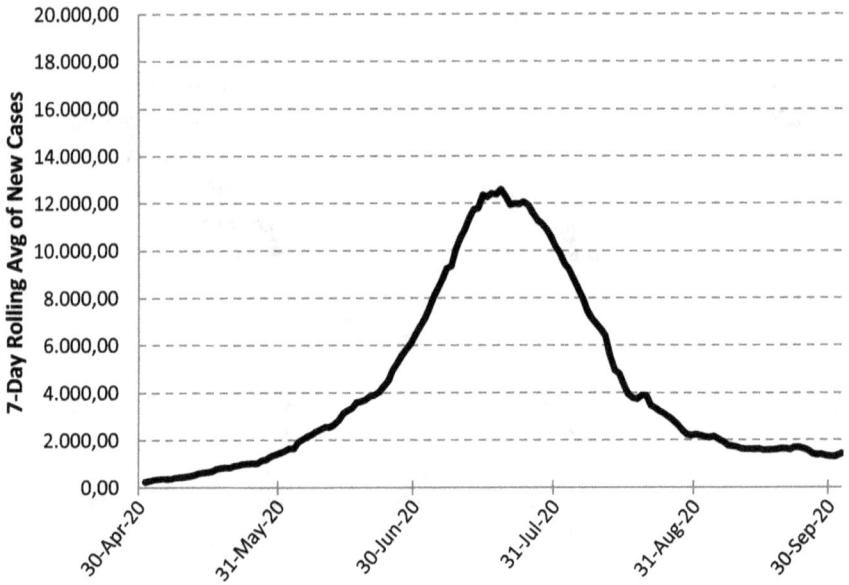

Graph 4.12: Daily confirmed COVID-19 in South Africa April–September 2020. Source of data: https://ourworldindata.org/

hypothesize that early lockdown followed by premature opening up may have two consequences. The first is of waves of longer duration; the second is that early lockdown may also precipitate lockdown fatigue, which results in non-compliance with lockdown measures and may inevitably increase a wave's duration.

Comparatively analyzing the vaccination rollout

Throughout the timelines we noted when countries started with their vaccine rollouts. This section closes the chapter by comparing the evolution of this, noting some stark differences between states.

Before turning to some of the rollout data, it is important to note how different political systems directly financed pharmaceutical companies to develop, manufacture, and distribute vaccine and treatments to fight COVID-19.

For example, the European Commission, acting on behalf of EU member states, 'financed a part of the upfront costs faced by vaccine producers from the €2.7 billion Emergency Support Instrument'[34] specially developed to deal with the pandemic. Beyond this, different member states individually gave funds to pharma companies such as BioNTech, which received to the tune of €375 million from the German government.[35] In the case of the Oxford/AstraZeneca vaccine, the UK government is similarly reported to have given around GBP 38.8 million towards the vaccine's development.[36]

Most impressively, through Operation Warp Speed, the US awarded more than $12 billion directly to key pharmaceutical firms by October 2020. These include: Pfizer/BioNTech, $1.95 billion; AstraZeneca, $1.2 bn; Johnson & Johnson, $1.5 bn; Moderna, $2.5 bn; and Novavax, $1.6 bn.[37] There was obviously some risk in doing this given that investment was made well before the vaccines had obtained regulatory approval.[38] Nonetheless, the potential benefits of developing vaccine(s) that would eventually gain regulatory approval outweighed the costs of having no preventive measure against COVID-19.

With this in mind, along with the information in Chapter 3 on the differences found globally regarding APCs, we can better understand some of the observations on the share of people vaccinated globally as of early May 2021. Graph 4.13 captures the percentages in the countries we have examined in this Chapter (plus the UK) that are vaccinated with either one or two doses as of May 9, 2021.

---

34 For more details on the EU's vaccine strategy, please see: https://ec.europa.eu/info/live-work-travel-eu/coronavirus-response/public-health/eu-vaccines-strategy_en

35 This was given days before results of Phase 3 clinical trials results were announced. See: https://www.biospace.com/article/biontech-receives-375-million-grant-from-german-federal-ministry-of-education-and-research/

36 To see the other public funders beyond the UK government, please see: https://www.theguardian.com/science/2021/apr/15/oxfordastrazeneca-covid-vaccine-research-was-97-publicly-funded

37 This is based on figures reported by Bloomberg in late October 2020: https://www.bloomberg.com/news/features/2020-10-29/inside-operation-warp-speed-s-18-billion-sprint-for-a-vaccine

38 This is an important point because billions were invested by the summer of 2020, several months before regulatory approval would take place. See: https://www.cnbc.com/2020/08/14/the-us-has-already-invested-billions-on-potential-coronavirus-vaccines-heres-where-the-deals-stand.html. In some cases, these investments with taxpayers' dollars saw limited immediate return. This is seen in the case of Sanofi and GSK that announced a delay to its COVID-19 vaccine program in December 2020, after having received $2.1 billion in July 2020. On the original funding received, please see: https://www.fiercepharma.com/pharma/sanofi-gsk-win-hefty-2-1b-operation-warp-speed-funding-for-covid-19-vaccine. For more information on the reasons for the delay, see the press release at: https://www.gsk.com/en-gb/media/press-releases/sanofi-and-gsk-announce-a-delay-in-their-adjuvanted-recombinant-protein-based-covid-19-vaccine-programme-to-improve-immune-response-in-the-elderly/

■ Share of people fully vaccinated   ■ Share of people only partly vaccinated against COVID-19

UK	26%	26%
US	34%	11%
Chile	37%	7.4%
Canada	3.3%	36%
Germany	9.4%	23%
Ireland	10%	17%
India	2.5%	7.2%
NZ	2.3%	3%
SA	0.7%	0%

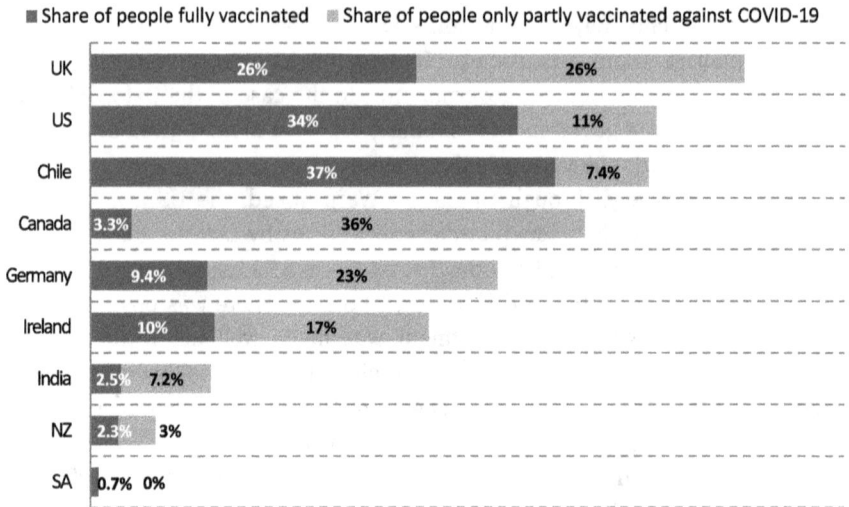

Graph 4.13: Percentage vaccinated against COVID-19, May 9, 2021. Source of data: https://our worldindata.org/

It shows that those states, such as the US and the UK, that generously funded pharmaceuticals have the highest percentages of those vaccinated. As seen in the US, a majority of those received two doses, which resulted in many seeing the US as vaccine 'hoarders'.[39] Interestingly, Chile also ranks relatively high given the preferential deal it was able to carve out with Pfizer/BioNTech and Sinovac.[40]

In contrast to the US, Canada has a lower percentage vaccinated, where a majority of those received only one dose. This is reflective of the country's initial approach to vaccinate more people with one dose in order to spread the vaccines available as widely as possible amongst the population (i.e. redistribute as equally as possible).[41]

Similar dynamics can be seen in Germany and Ireland, which were also seeing initial shortfalls of vaccines given that some companies had not delivered on

---

39 See: https://fortune.com/2021/04/04/us-vaccine-hoarding-nationalism-diplomacy-china-rus sia-india/

40 For more on developments in Chile, including an increase in surges in 2021 given the premature loosening of lockdown in the wake of vaccination, see: https://www.scientificamerican. com/article/reckless-rush-to-reopen-threatens-chiles-exemplary-vaccination-strategy/

41 See: https://www.macleans.ca/news/how-soon-are-second-doses-coming-for-canadians-and-who-will-get-them-first/

numbers agreed with the European Commission as discussed in the previous chapter.

Notwithstanding, European rates are still much higher than those in India and South Africa, where less than 10% and only 1% of their population have received vaccines, respectively. New Zealand has been criticized for its slow vaccine rollout, which may just be a 'recipe for disaster' for a country that witnessed a comparatively robust response to COVID-19 when there was no medical solution as the start of the chapter examined.[42]

Conclusions

This chapter analyzed policy developments during COVID-19, assessing significant countries' performance against the typology developed in Chapter 3. We summarized these developments by constructing timelines, showing key policies formulated during the four different phases. It is important to note that while the typology itself represents an objective benchmark against which one can assess what countries did at what time during the pandemic, it was not our objective to claim that some states did it 'better' or 'worse' than others *per se*. Rather, in our discussion we broadly outlined two types of country timelines that could be theoretically expected: those that resembled a 'layer cake' demonstrating that states pursued the policies that were expected of them in each phase as per our typology, in contrast to a 'marble cake' which showed that policies expected in some phases were formulated in others.

The evidence demonstrated that:
- New Zealand, ostensibly the only country in our analysis that clearly sought to eliminate the virus (as opposed to simply live with it) while making evidenced-based policy decisions, saw a timeline that was most representative of a layer cake.
- This was also seen in Germany as well as in Canada, which in contrast to its US neighbor had a more clear, centralized plan to deal with COVID-19.
- Other countries which sought to live with the virus, most notably Ireland (in the 2nd and 3rd waves), had timelines representative of marble cakes. The Irish opened up in Christmas 2020 when they should have been pursuing policies to control the virus.

---

42 See: https://edition.cnn.com/2021/04/15/asia/new-zealand-australia-covid-vaccine-intl-dst-hnk/index.html

- This marble cake was similarly seen in India, South Africa and Chile in their first wave, all of which pursued lockdown policies sooner than expected, while later opening up sooner than expected.

We now turn to the main takeaways from the book, and lessons to be taken from the study.

Chapter 5
Conclusions

This book has brought together a novel cross-interdisciplinary investigation from both natural and social sciences, representing a true hybrid across disciplines by examining both the 'science' and 'politics' of pandemics. By first considering the dynamics surrounding viruses, proposed vaccines, and antiviral therapies, we contextualize a policy framework for what should be done by countries in a pandemic and then examined what governments actually did during the COVID-19 crisis.

In more detail, the objective of Chapter 2 was to overview viruses, pandemics, vaccines and antiviral treatments (both small-molecule and biologics). Here we described the structure and replication of viruses, the history of previous pandemics, the disease stages of COVID-19, and the most important variants reported for SARS-CoV-2. We then turned to describe the processes of drug and vaccine development as well as the proposed drugs to treat the disease and vaccines to prevent it. Its contribution to the literature was to offer a succinct summary of key scientific ideas. This is of particular value to social science scholars seeking to understand the science behind viruses (as well as how to treat and prevent them), thereby allowing for better evaluation of public policies taken by governments during a viral pandemic and of how much scientific knowledge actually shapes policy-makers' decisions. The evidence presented allows for a clear understanding of why, in the absence of a scientific solution to deal with a viral pandemic, public policy choices are paramount.

The objective of Chapter 3 was thus to develop a typology of what countries need to do, when, and why during a pandemic. This classification scheme can be used by anyone, in any country, during any pandemic. Here we outlined a strong and focused set of policies during the four phases of a pandemic: anticipating and early virus detection; containing the virus when first cases are detected; controlling and mitigating the spread of the virus; and opening up society when there is reduced transmission. By developing this four-phased typology, a main contribution is to offer a clear policy roadmap that guides countries during the different stages of a pandemic they may find themselves in, which is necessary in order to transcend the indecisiveness of governments that was demonstrated during COVID-19. The classification scheme also informs states of how to implement a feedback mechanism during the four phases, which is of particular salience given the variants and potential new strains of COVID-19 that may render vaccine or anti-viral treatments ineffective in the future.

https://doi.org/10.1515/9783110743609-006

The aim of Chapter 4 was to examine policies pursued in key states found worldwide during COVID-19, assessing their performance against expectations in our typology. A main contribution here is that it represents one of the first attempts to date to comparatively analyze developments across the globe during any pandemic using the same objective benchmark, namely, the classification scheme developed in Chapter 3. The visualizations in the chapter highlighted clearly, yet simply, those political systems which pursued policies in a way that was consistent with our typology and those that did not, respectively reflected in having timelines that mostly resembled a structure akin to either a 'layer cake', or a 'marble cake'.

There are several lessons to be drawn from this investigation. From a natural science perspective, there are at least three:

- Understanding how a virus replicates and spreads is significant because the spread of viruses and their replication cycle are unique to each viral family. Dealing with new pandemics requires a deep understanding of this in order to identify targets for the development of therapies and vaccines.
- Understanding the stages involved in the development and regulatory controls of drugs and vaccines is important, given that this is a complex process that requires time and resources. While vaccines against COVID-19 were developed in a relatively short amount of time, several other viral diseases have been less fortunate. Even with variants and potential strains of COVID-19 on the horizon, countries must keep vigilant and continue to fund R&D to deal with such scenarios. Furthermore, there are several people who may not be able to use vaccines, so it is important to develop antiviral treatments that require a long process of discovery and development.
- To overcome the issues associated with drug and vaccine development, stronger investment in R&D would accelerate not only the discovery of treatment and prevention agents, but also the development of faster and more efficient detection technologies.

From a social science perspective, there are at least three key lessons:

- What governments formulate makes a difference, and it is important to take a holistic approach. Our analysis outlined and demonstrated the importance of several public policies that states should pursue in the absence of a vaccine or antiviral treatments. This ranges from health, economic, social, regulatory, as well as science and technology policies, all of which interplay in the various phases. No one policy area is more important than another, and it is important that states take a 'big picture' policy approach when formulating what needs to be done, when and why. Considering how difficult it is to develop drugs and vaccines, it is important to formulate and coordinate a variety of policy areas before scientific solutions are found.

– Domestic level governance needs to embrace a new way of thinking. A new, structured way of thinking need to be harnessed by national governments in order to more fully understand and then deal with viral threats, especially for those for which there is no immediate medical solution. While our typology offers a guide to help governments in this process, it is still up to them to prioritize changing the way they think: they need to get ready to act even before the next pandemic happens by earmarking resources towards that now, particularly towards R&D. In this regard, analysis by Mazey and Richardson (2020) is absolutely key – even states like New Zealand which handled COVID-19 well (to date), failed to fully engage in anticipatory politics beforehand.

– The international level needs to embrace a harmonized approach. There are two dimensions to this.

   – In the first, our study demonstrated the clear variation of government policies pursued throughout the different phases and waves during COVID-19. One lesson to prevent this disparate approach in the future is having more harmonization. This may be best achieved by giving the institutions at the international level, such as the WHO, a leading and decisive role given their knowledge of how the virus is replicating and spreading globally. To this end our typology can help the international level to develop a policy plan that can then be transposed from one level of governance to another.

   – In a second dimension, more specifically for COVID-19 and for future pandemics where there is a vaccine solution, there needs to be a global rollout plan. We have clearly seen the different speeds of vaccine distribution throughout the globe. Delays in distribution across the world facilitate mutations, meaning that treatments developed may be rendered less effective over time, sowing the seeds for the next pandemic. Protecting everyone protects us all.

Using our typology as a guide, future research may consider more fully the dynamics between public and private actors when policy is made during a pandemic. For example, our research showed the significance of border restrictions throughout the various phases in our typology, as seen in our analysis of flight data. Future researchers may consider the interactions between public actors (such as politicians, regulators and civil servants) and private actors (lobbyists from the airline sector and civil society actors) when developing this policy and examine whether or not scientific criteria guided and played a role during policy deliberation. Another example stemming from our investigation would be to fully examine the vaccines/antiviral therapies that have been developed by the different Pharma companies during COVID-19, and then analyze acquisition of these therapies/vaccines by governments. The 'science' side of the project would thus examine in detail the treatments developed by the companies, while the 'social science' side would examine the role of these same companies in lobbying for state research funds to develop their products as well as secure lucrative advance purchase agreements.

Performing such investigation would extend upon the interdisciplinary approach to research that we have striven for in this book.

Appendix A
Supplemental information
on methods of analysis

As discussed in Chapter 4, this study relies on a mixed method approach when trying to capture the various policies/strategies pursued by states in the different phases, as per the typology developed. Below we consider the main sources that are used to measure when the phases start and end for each country as well as the policies that states pursued.

Phase 1: Anticipating and early detection

The anticipation and early detection phase should have started shortly after the virus was detected in Wuhan and when the WHO declared COVID-19 a public emergency on January 30, 2020.

The concepts outlined in the typology and how they are measured, which are then presented in the timelines seen in Chapter 4, are as follows:

Concept	Method of analysis/Measurement
States define problem and develop Initial Emergency Action Plan	We examine any government statements released at the central government level as well as documents available on websites such as https://covid19policywatch.org/. We also considered data on the Oxford Covid-19 Government Response Tracker (OxCGRT) database (https://www.bsg.ox.ac.uk/research/research-projects/covid-19-government-response-tracker), analysis of Code H4 (Emergency Investment in Healthcare; also examined for Phase 2)
Pursuing regulatory policies of restricting/ monitoring movements on international borders.	Analysis of information available on the CAPA Aviation Database (https://centreforaviation.com/data). Analysis of OxCGRT C8 (Restrictions on External Movement)
Start with public information campaigns	Analysis of government press releases, newspaper reports, and OxCGRT H1 (Presence of public information campaigns)

https://doi.org/10.1515/9783110743609-007

Phase 2: Strategies to contain the virus

The start of Phase 2 theoretically takes place when the first confirmed cases are detected in the country. Our World in Data, an authoritative freely available database that has collected information for all countries worldwide by compiling data from leading sources (such as the CDC, ECDC and Johns Hopkins University CSSE COVID-19 Data), allows us to establish when Phase 2 for all states should have started by simply seeing when the first cases were recorded.

The sources and indicators relied on to measure the various concepts outlined in Phase 2, again both qualitative and quantitative in nature, are as follows:

Concept	Method of analysis/Measurement
Testing, contract tracing and isolation of all population	Analysis of government documents and secondary literature, examining state initiatives to localize quarantine of suspected cases; OxCGRT database Code H2 (Testing Policy), H3 (Contact Tracing)
Continue with information campaign, to minimize 'infodemic'	Analysis of government documents, newspaper reports, OxCGRT, H1 (Presence of public information campaigns)
Developing regulatory policies on restricting movement internationally	Analysis of information available on the CAPA Aviation Database (https://centreforaviation.com/data). We were particularly interested in seeing the change in traffic from major airports as a strategy to contain the virus.
Starting initiatives to promote R&D	Government announcements on funding schemes as well as information from https://covid19policywatch.org/

Phase 3: Policies to control and mitigate the virus

We demonstrate an initial surge in the number of cases, meaning a sharp or sudden rise in cases followed by either sustained or exponential growth, by examining the 7-day rolling average of cases in Our World in Data. This indicates when Phase 3 policies should have started. This measurement is also used when trying to determine when states enter into Phase 3 again in the case there are second waves.

Secondly, we measure the state's policy responses in Phase 3 by considering various indicators to measure efforts regarding lockdown, health and economic policies using qualitative and quantitative evidence as follows.

Concept	Method of analysis/Measurement
Lockdown policies	Analysis of government documents and secondary literature, including articles and newspaper reports; CAPA Aviation Database; OxCGRT database, codes on: closing schools (C1), working from/staying at home (C2&C6), canceling public events and restriction on gatherings (C3&C4), closing public transport (C5), internal travel restrictions (C7).
Economic policies to deal with job losses, household relief, economic stimulus	OxCGRT database, analysis of: E1 (measuring income support for those losing jobs; ordinal); E2 (measuring if government freezes financial obligations); E3 (measuring the economic stimulus policies adopted). To gain a solid overview, analysis was also made of government documents (particularly those from Ministries of Economy and/or Finance, or equivalent), relevant information from civil society organizations and NGOs, newspaper reports, and academic literature.
Social policies	As there are several policies that could have been examined, given space limitations we specifically examined *housing policy*, with a focus on initiatives states pursued with regard to preventing evictions during the pandemic. This information was primarily collected from government announcements as well as https://covid19policy watch.org/

Phase 4: Opening up and eradicating the virus

This phase should have taken place theoretically when there were clear indications that it was safe to do so once the virus was controlled and mitigated. This is measured by seeing when the number of cases plateaued (i.e. flattened), with case numbers ideally being at zero, and we will ascertain this by examining the 7-day rolling average of new confirmed cases found in Our World in Data.

Sources mentioned above are examined for reversal of lockdown, while government sources are also to be examined to determine lifting lockdown and contingency plans, if any. Information from Our World in Data is used to demonstrate the comparative differences when the vaccine rollout started.

Bibliography

Addo, P. C., Jiaming, F., Kulbo, N. B., & Liangqiang, L. (2020). COVID-19: fear appeal favoring purchase behavior towards personal protective equipment. *The Service Industries Journal*, 40(7 – 8), pp. 471 – 490. Available at: https://doi.org/10.1080/02642069.2020. 1751823

Ali, M., Nelson, A. R., Lopez, A. L. , Sack, D. A. (2015). Updated global burden of cholera in endemic countries. *PLOS Neglected Tropical Diseases*, 9(6), p. e0003832. Available at: https://doi.org/10.1371/journal.pntd.0003832

Andersen, K.G., Rambaut, A., Lipkin, W.I., Holmes, E. C. & Garry, R.F. (2020). The proximal origin of SARS-CoV-2. *Nature Medicine*, 26, pp. 450 – 452. Available at: https://doi.org/ 10.1038/s41591-020-0820-9

Anderson, R. M., Heesterbeek, H., Klinkenberg, D., & Hollingsworth, T. D. (2020). How will country-based mitigation measures influence the course of the COVID-19 epidemic?. *The Lancet*, 395(10228), pp. 931 – 934. Available at: https://doi.org/10.1016/S0140-6736(20) 30567-5

Balmford, B., Annan, J. D., Hargreaves, J. C., Altoè, M., & Bateman, I. J. (2020). Cross-country comparisons of COVID-19: Policy, politics and the price of life. *Environmental and Resource Economics*, 76(4), pp. 525 – 551. Available at: https://doi.org/10.1007/s10640-020-00466-5

Baraniuk, C. (2021). Covid-19: What do we know about Sputnik V and other Russian vaccines?. *BMJ*, 372(1), p. n743. Available at: https://doi.org/10.1136/bmj.n743

Baris, O. F., & Pelizzo, R. (2020). Research Note: Governance Indicators Explain Discrepancies in COVID-19 Data. *World Affairs*, 183(3), pp. 216 – 234. Available at: https://doi.org/10. 1177/0043820020945683

Béland, D., & Marier, P. (2020). COVID-19 and long-term care policy for older people in Canada. *Journal of Aging & Social Policy*, 32(4 – 5), pp. 358 – 364. Available at: https:// doi.org/10.1080/08959420.2020.1764319

Berkowitz, R. L., Gao, X., Michaels, E. K., & Mujahid, M. S. (2020). Structurally vulnerable neighbourhood environments and racial/ethnic COVID-19 inequities. *Cities & Health*. Available at: https://doi.org/10.1080/23748834.2020.1792069

Blouin Genest, G., Burlone, N., Champagne, E., Eastin, C., & Ogaranko, C. (2021). Translating COVID-19 emergency plans into policy: A comparative analysis of three Canadian provinces. *Policy Design and Practice*, 4(1), pp. 115 – 132. Available at: https://doi.org/10. 1080/25741292.2020.1868123

Blum, S., & Dobrotić, I. (2021). Childcare-policy responses in the COVID-19 pandemic: unpacking cross-country variation. *European Societies*, 23(sup1), S545-S563. Available at: https://doi.org/10.1080/14616696.2020.1831572

Bos, K., Harkins, K., Herbig, A., Coscolla, M., Weber, N., Comas, I., Forrest, S.A., Bryant, J. M., Harris, S. R., Schuenemann, V. J., Campbell, T. J., Majander, K., Wilbur, A. K., Guichon, R. A., Wolfe Steadman, D. L., Collins Cook, D., Niemann, S. Behr, M. A., Zumarraga, M., Bastida, R., Huson, D., Nieselt, K., Young, D., Parkhill, J., Buikstra, J. E., Gagneux, S. Stone, A. C. and Krause, J., (2014). Pre-Columbian mycobacterial genomes reveal seals as a source of New World human tuberculosis. *Nature,* 514(1), pp. 494 – 497. Available at: https://doi.org/10.1038/nature13591

https://doi.org/10.1515/9783110743609-008

Butowt, R., Bilinska, K., & Von Bartheld, C. S. (2020). Chemosensory dysfunction in COVID-19: Integration of genetic and epidemiological data points to D614G spike protein variant as a contributing factor. *ACS chemical neuroscience*, 11(20), pp. 3180–3184. Available at: https://doi.org/10.1021/acschemneuro.0c00596

Boudjema, S., Finance, J., Coulibaly, F., Meddeb, L., Tissot-Dupont, H., Michel, M., Lagier, J. C., Million, M., Radulesco, T., Michel, J., Brouqui, P., Raoult, D., Fenollar, F., & Parola, P. (2020). Olfactory and gustative disorders for the diagnosis of COVID-19. *Travel medicine and infectious disease*, 37(1), p. 101875. Available at: https://doi.org/10.1016/j.tmaid.2020.101875

Cao, B., Wang, Y., Wen, D., Liu, W., Wang, J., Fan, G., Ruan, L., Song, B., Cai, Y., Wei, M., Li, X., Xia, J., Chen, N., Xiang, J., Yu, T., Bai, T., Xie, X., Zhang, L., Li, C., Yuan, Y., Chen, H., Li, H., Huang, H., Tu, S., Gong, F., Liu, Y., Wei, Y., Dong, C., Zhou, F., Gu, X., Xu, J., Liu, Z., Zhang, Y., Li, H., Shang, L., Wang, K., Li, K., Zhou, X., Dong, X., Qu, Z., Lu, S., Hu, X., Ruan, S., Luo, S., Wu, J., Peng, L., Cheng, F., Pan, L., Zou, J., Jia, C., Wang, J., Liu, X., Wang, S., Wu, X., Ge, Q., He, J., Zhan, H., Qiu, F., Guo, L., Huang, C., Jaki, T., Hayden, F. G., Horby P. W., Zhang, D., & Wang, C. (2020). A trial of lopinavir–ritonavir in adults hospitalized with severe Covid-19. *New England journal of medicine*, 382(19), pp. 1787–1799. Available at: https://doi.org/10.1056/NEJMoa2001282

Capano, G. (2020). Policy design and state capacity in the COVID-19 emergency in Italy: If you are not prepared for the (un) expected, you can be only what you already are. *Policy and Society*, 39(3), pp. 326–344. Available at: https://doi.org/10.1080/14494035.2020.1783790

Carpenter, D., & Dunn, J. (2021). We're All Teachers Now: Remote Learning During COVID-19. *Journal of School Choice*, 14(4), pp. 567–594. Available at: https://doi.org/10.1080/15582159.2020.1822727

Cepaluni, G., Dorsch, M., & Branyiczki, R. (2020). Political regimes and deaths in the early stages of the COVID-19 pandemic. 27th of April. Available at SSRN: https://dx.doi.org/10.2139/ssrn.3586767

Chand, M., Hopkins, S., Dabrera, G., Achison, C., Barclay, W., Ferguson, N., Volz, E., Loman, N., Rambaut, A., Barrett, J. (2020). *Investigation of novel SARS-COV-2 variant: Variant of Concern 202012/01*. London: Public Health England. Available at: https://assets.publishing.service.gov.uk/government/uploads/system/uploads/attachment_data/file/959438/Technical_Briefing_VOC_SH_NJL2_SH2.pdf

Chari, R. (2015). *Life After Privatization*. Oxford: Oxford University Press.

Chari, R., & Bernhagen, P. (2011). Financial and economic crisis: explaining the sunset over the Celtic Tiger. *Irish Political Studies*, 26(4), pp. 473–488. Available at: https://doi.org/10.1080/07907184.2011.619736

Chari, R., & Heywood, P. M. (2009). Analysing the policy process in democratic Spain. *West European Politics*, 32(1), pp. 26–54. Available at: https://doi.org/10.1080/01402380802509800

Chari, R., Hogan, J., Murphy, G., & Crepaz, M. (2010). *Regulating lobbying: a global comparison*, 1st ed. Manchester: Manchester University Press.

Chari, R., Hogan, J., Murphy, G., & Crepaz, M. (2019). *Regulating lobbying: a global comparison*, 2nd ed. Manchester: Manchester University Press.

Chari, R & Kritzinger, S. (2006). *Understanding EU Policy Making*. London: Pluto Press.

Chopera, D. (2020). Can Africa withstand COVID-19? *Project Syndicate.* 24th of March. Available at: https://www.project-syndicate.org

Cifuentes-Faura, J. (2021). Analysis of containment measures and economic policies arising from COVID-19 in the European Union. *International Review of Applied Economics*, 35(2), pp. 242–255. Available at: https://doi.org/10.1080/02692171.2020.1864300

Crepaz, M. & G. Arikan (2021). Information disclosure and political trust during the COVID-19 crisis: experimental evidence from Ireland. *Journal of Elections, Public Opinion and Parties, 31*(s1): 96–108. Available at: https://doi.org/10.1080/17457289.2021.1924738

Collier, D., LaPorte, J., & Seawright, J. (2012). Putting typologies to work: Concept formation, measurement, and analytic rigor. *Political Research Quarterly*, 65(1), pp. 217–232. Available at: https://doi.org/10.1177%2F1065912912437162

Crawford, D. H. (2018). *Viruses: a very short introduction.* Oxford: Oxford University Press.

Creech, C. B., Walker, S. C., & Samuels, R. J. (2021). SARS-CoV-2 vaccines. *Jama*, 325(13), pp. 1318–1320. Available at: https://doi.org/10.1001/jama.2021.3199

Crepaz, M., & Arikan, G. (2021). Information disclosure and political trust during the COVID-19 crisis: experimental evidence from Ireland. *Journal of Elections, Public Opinion and Parties*, 31(sup1), pp. 96–108. Available at: https://doi.org/10.1080/17457289.2021. 1924738

Czypionka, T. & Reiss, M. (2021). "Three approaches to handling the Covid-19 crisis in federal countries: Germany, Austria and Switzerland" in Greer, S. L., King, E. J., Massard da Fonseca, E., & Perlata-Santos, A. (eds.) *Coronavirus politics: the comparative politics and policy of Covid-19.* Ann Arbor: University of Michigan Press, pp. 295–319.

Davidovitz, M., Cohen, N., & Gofen, A. (2021). Governmental Response to Crises and Its Implications for Street-Level Implementation: Policy Ambiguity, Risk, and Discretion during the COVID-19 Pandemic. *Journal of Comparative Policy Analysis: Research and Practice*, 23(1), pp. 120–130. Available at: https://doi.org/10.1080/13876988.2020. 1841561

Davies, N. G., Jarvis, C. I., CMMID COVID-19 Working Group, Edmunds, W. J., Jewell, N. P., Diaz-Ordaz, K., & Keogh, R. H. (2021). Increased mortality in community-tested cases of SARS-CoV-2 lineage B. 1.1. 7. *Nature*, 593(1), pp. 270–274. Available at: https://doi.org/ 10.1038/s41586-021-03426-1 3

Davis, M. (2019). 'Uncertainty and immunity in public communications on pandemics', in Bjorkdahl, K. & Carlsen, B. (eds.), *Pandemics, Publics and Politics.* London: Palgrave, pp. 29–42. Available at: https://dx.doi.org/10.1007%2F978-981-13-2802-2_3

Dean, N. (2020). 'Steps to a Better COVID-19 response' in Boston Review (ed.). *Thinking in a Pandemic: the Crisis of Science and Policy in the age of COVID-19.* Cambridge: Verso Books, pp. 147–156.

Delanty, G. (2021). 'Introduction: The Pandemic in Historical and Global Context' in G. Delanty (ed.), *Pandemics, Politics, and Society* (Berlin: De Gruyter), 1–21

Devakumar, D., Shannon, G., Bhopal, S. & Abubakar, I. (2020). Racism and discrimination in COVID-19 responses. *Lancet*, 395(10231) p. 1194. Available at: https://doi.org/10.1016/ S0140-6736(20)30792-3

De Waal, A. (2020). 'New Pathogen, Old Politics', in Boston Review (ed.). *Thinking in a Pandemic: the Crisis of Science and Policy in the age of COVID-19.* Cambridge: Verso Books, pp. 10–48.

Di Moia, J. P. (2020). Contact Tracing and COVID-19: The South Korean Context for Public Health Enforcement. *East Asian Science, Technology and Society: An International Journal*, 14(4), pp. 657–665. Available at: https://doi.org/10.1215/18752160-8771448

Dunlop, C. A., Ongaro, E., & Baker, K. (2020). Researching COVID-19: A research agenda for public policy and administration scholars. *Public Policy and Administration*, 35(4), pp. 365–383. Available at: https://doi.org/10.1177%2F0952076720939631

Eftekhari, A., Alipour, M., Chodari, L., Maleki Dizaj, S., Ardalan, M. R., Samiei, M., Sharifi, S., Zununi Vahed, S., Huseynova, I., Khalilov, R., Ahmadian, E., & Cucchiarini, M. (2021). A comprehensive review of detection methods for SARS-CoV-2. Microorganisms, 9(2), p. 232. Available at: https://doi.org/10.3390/microorganisms9020232

El Masri, A., & Sabzalieva, E. (2020). Dealing with disruption, rethinking recovery: Policy responses to the COVID-19 pandemic in higher education. *Policy Design and Practice*, 3(3), pp. 312–333. Available at: https://doi.org/10.1080/25741292.2020.1813359

Ertan, D., El-Hage, W., Thierrée, S., Javelot, H., & Hingray, C. (2020). COVID-19: urgency for distancing from domestic violence. *European journal of psychotraumatology*, 11(1), p. 1800245. Available at: https://doi.org/10.1080/20008198.2020.1800245

Fafard, P., Cassola, A., MacAulay, M. & Palkovits, M. (2021). "The politics and policy of Canada's Covid-19 response" in Greer, S. L., King, E. J., Massard da Fonseca, E., & Perlata-Santos, A. (eds.) *Coronavirus politics: the comparative politics and policy of Covid-19*. Ann Arbor: University of Michigan Press, pp. 459–477.

Fehr A.R. & Perlman S. (2015). Coronaviruses: An Overview of Their Replication and Pathogenesis, in Maier H., Bickerton, E. & Britton P. (eds.) *Coronaviruses: Methods and Protocols*. Methods in Molecular Biology, 1282. New York: Humana Press. Available at: https://doi.org/10.1007/978-1-4939-2438-7_1

Feng, W., Newbigging, A. M., Le, C., Pang, B., Peng, H., Cao, Y., Wu, J., Abbas, G., Song, J., Wang, D.-B., Cui, M., Tao, J., Tyrrell, D. L., Zhang, X.-E., Zhang, H., & Le, X. C. (2020). Molecular diagnosis of COVID-19: challenges and research needs. *Analytical Chemistry*, 92(15), pp. 10196–10209. Available at: https://doi.org/10.1021/acs.analchem.0c02060

Fineberg, H. V. (2014). Pandemic preparedness and response—lessons from the H1N1 influenza of 2009. *New England Journal of Medicine*, 370(14), pp. 1335–1342. Available at: https://doi.org/10.1056/NEJMra1208802

Fong, M.W., Gao, H., Wong, J. Y., Xiao, J., Shiu, E. Y. C., Ryu, S & Cowling, B. J. (2020). Nonpharmaceutical Measures for Pandemic Influenza in Nonhealthcare Settings: Social Distancing Measures. *Emerging Infectious Diseases*, 26(5), pp. 976–984. Available at: https://doi.org/10.3201/eid2605.190995

Fuller, J. (2020). 'From Pandemic Facts to Pandemic Policies' in Boston Review (ed.). *Thinking in a Pandemic: the Crisis of Science and Policy in the age of COVID-19*. Cambridge: Verso Books. pp. 107–117.

Gautret, P., Million, M., Jarrot, P. A., Camoin-Jau, L., Colson, P., Fenollar, F., Leone, M., La Scola, B., Devaux, C., Gaubert, J. Y., Mege, J.-L., Vitte, J., Melenotte, C., Rolain, J.-M., Parola, P., Lagier, J.-C., Brouqui, P. & Raoult, D. (2020). Natural history of COVID-19 and therapeutic options. *Expert Review of Clinical Immunology*, 16(12), pp. 1159–1184. Available at: https://doi.org/10.1080/1744666X.2021.1847640

Goldmann, M. (2020). Human rights and democracy in economic policy reform: the European COVID-19 response under scrutiny. *The International Journal of Human Rights*, 24(9), pp. 1290–1310. Available at: https://doi.org/10.1080/13642987.2020.1811697

Greinacher, A., Thiele, T., Warkentin, T. E., Weisser, K., Kyrle, P. A., & Eichinger, S. (2021). Thrombotic thrombocytopenia after ChAdOx1 nCov-19 vaccination. *New England Journal of Medicine*, 384(22), pp. 2092–2101. Available at: https://doi.org/10.1056/NEJ Moa2104840

Gunst, J. D., Staerke, N. B., Pahus, M. H., Kristensen, L. H., Bodilsen, J., Lohse, N., Dalgaard, L. S., Brønnum, D., Fröbert, O., Hønge, B., Johansen, I. S., Monrad, I., Erikstrup, C., Rosendal, R., Vilstrup, E., Mariager, T., Bove, D. G., Offersen, R., Shakar, S., Cajander, S., Jørgensen, N. P., Sritharan, S. S., Breining, P., Jespersen, S., Mortensen, K. L., Jensen, M. L., Kolte, L., Frattari, G. S., Larsen, C. S., Storgaard, M., Nielsen, L. P., Tolstrup, M., Sædder, E. A., Østergaard, L. J., Ngo, H. T. T., Jensen, M. H., Højen, J. F., Kjolby, M., & Søgaard, O. S. (2021). Efficacy of the TMPRSS2 inhibitor camostat mesilate in patients hospitalized with Covid-19-a double-blind randomized controlled trial. *EClinicalMedicine*, 35(1), p. 100849. Available at: https://doi.org/10.1016/j.eclinm.2021. 100849

Guo, Y. R., Cao, Q. D., Hong, Z. S., Tan, Y. Y., Chen, S. D., Jin, H. J., Tan, K. S., Wang, D. T. & Yan, Y. (2020). The origin, transmission and clinical therapies on coronavirus disease 2019 (COVID-19) outbreak–an update on the status. *Military Medical Research*, 7(11). Available at: https://doi.org/10.1186/s40779-020-00240-0

Hale, T., Angrist, N., Kira, B., Petherick, A., Phillips, T. & Webster, S. (2020a). "Variation in Government Responses to COVID-19" Version 6.0. *Blavatnik School of Government Working Paper*. 25th of May. Available at: www.bsg.ox.ac.uk/covidtracker

Hale T., Webster, S., Petherick, A., Phillips, T. & Kira, B. (2020b). Oxford COVID-19 Government Response Tracker. Blavatnik School of Government. Available at: www.bsg. ox.ac.uk/covidtracker

Hargreaves, J. R., & Logie, C. H. (2020). Lifting lockdown policies: A critical moment for COVID-19 stigma. *Global public health*, 15(12), pp. 1917–1923. Available at: https://doi. org/10.1080/17441692.2020.1825771

Harris, J. (2021). "Confronting legacies and charting a new course? The politics of Coronavirus response in South Africa" in Greer, S. L., King, E. J., Massard da Fonseca, E., & Perlata-Santos, A. (eds.) *Coronavirus politics: the comparative politics and policy of Covid-19*. Ann Arbor: University of Michigan Press, pp. 580–599.

Hartley, K., Bales, S., & Bali, A. S. (2021). COVID-19 response in a unitary state: emerging lessons from Vietnam. *Policy Design and Practice*, 4(1), pp. 152–168. Available at: https://doi.org/10.1080/25741292.2021.1877923

Hendy, S., Steyn, N., James, A., Plank, M. J., Hannah, K., Binny, R. N., & Lustig, A. (2021). Mathematical modelling to inform New Zealand's COVID-19 response. *Journal of the Royal Society of New Zealand*, 51(sup1), S86-S106. Available at: https://doi.org/10.1080/ 03036758.2021.1876111

Hershkovitz, I., Donoghue, H. D., Minnikin, D. E., Besra, G. S., Lee, O. Y, Gernaey, A. M., Galili, E., Eshed, V., Greenblatt, C. L., Lemma, E., Kahila Bar-Gal, G., Spigelman, M., (2008). PLOS ONE, 3(10), p. e3426. Available at: https://doi.org/10.1371/journal.pone. 0003426

Hodcroft, E. B., Zuber, M., Nadeau, S., Vaughan, T.G., Crawford, K. H. D., Althaus, C. L., Reichmuth, M. L., Bowen, J. E., Walls, A. C., Corti, D., Bloom, J. D., Veesler, D., Mateo, D., Hernando, A., Comas, I., & González Candelas, F., SeqCOVID-SPAIN consortium,

Stadler, T. & Neher, R. A. (2020). *MedRxiv*, Preprint. Available at: https://doi.org/10.1101/2020.10.25.20219063

Hoffmann, M., Kleine-Weber, H., Schroeder, S., Krüger, N., Herrler, T., Erichsen, S., Tobias, S. S., Herrler, G., Wu, N., Nitsche, A., Müller, M. A., Drosten, C. & Pöhlmann, S. (2020a). SARS-CoV-2 cell entry depends on ACE2 and TMPRSS2 and is blocked by a clinically proven protease inhibitor. *Cell*, 181(2), pp. 271–280. Available at: https://doi.org/10.1016/j.cell.2020.02.052

Hoffmann, M., Schroeder, S., Kleine-Weber, H., Müller, M. A., Drosten, C., & Pöhlmann, S. (2020b). Nafamostat mesylate blocks activation of SARS-CoV-2: new treatment option for COVID-19. *Antimicrobial agents and chemotherapy*, 64(6), p. e00754–20. Available at: https://doi.org/10.1128/AAC.00754-20

Honigsbaum, M. (2020). *The Pandemic Century: A History of Global Contagion from the Spanish Flu to Covid-19*. London: WH Allen.

Horton, R. (2020). *The COVID-19 Catastrophe: What's Gone Wrong and How To Stop It Happening Again*. Cambridge: Polity.

Hossain, M. P., Junus, A., Zhu, X., Jia, P., Wen, T., Pfeiffer, D. & Yuan, H. (2020). The effects of border control and quarantine measures on the spread of COVID-19. *Epidemics*, 32(1), p. 100397. Available at: https://doi.org/10.1016/j.epidem.2020.100397

Ioannidis, J. (2020). 'The Totality of Evidence' in *Thinking in a Pandemic: the Crisis of Science and Policy in the age of COVID-19*. Cambridge: Verso Books. pp. 100–106.

Kelly-Cirino, C. D., Nkengasong, J., Kettler, H., Tongio, I., Gay-Andrieu, F., Escadafal, C., Piot, P., Peeling, R. W., Gadde, R. & Boehme, C. (2019). Importance of diagnostics in epidemic and pandemic preparedness. *BMJ global health*, 4(Suppl 2), p. 001179. Available at: http://dx.doi.org/10.1136/bmjgh-2018-001179

Kettl, D. F. (2020). States Divided: The Implications of American Federalism for Covid-19. *Public Administration Review*, 80(4), pp. 595–602. Available at: https://doi.org/10.1111/puar.13243

Klingberg, T. (2020). More than viral: outsiders, Others, and the illusions of COVID-19. *Eurasian Geography and Economics*, 61(4–5), pp. 362–373. Available at: https://doi.org/10.1080/15387216.2020.1799833

Kowarz, E., Krutzke, L., Reis, J., Bracharz, S., Kochanek, S., & Marschalek, R. (2021). "Vaccine-Induced Covid-19 Mimicry" Syndrome:Splice reactions within the SARS-CoV-2 Spike open reading frame result in Spike protein variants that may cause thromboembolic events in patients immunized with vector-based vaccines. Preprint, *Research Square*, 1. Available at: https://doi.org/10.21203/rs.3.rs-558954/v1

Ladi, S., & Tsarouhas, D. (2020). EU economic governance and Covid-19: policy learning and windows of opportunity. *Journal of European Integration*, 42(8), pp. 1041–1056. Available at: https://doi.org/10.1080/07036337.2020.1852231

Lee, S., Hwang, C., & Moon, M. J. (2020). Policy learning and crisis policy-making: quadruple-loop learning and COVID-19 responses in South Korea. *Policy and Society*, 39(3), pp. 363–381. Available at: https://doi.org/10.1080/14494035.2020.1785195

Li, Y., & Galea, S. (2020). Racism and the COVID-19 epidemic: recommendations for health care workers. *American Journal of Public Health*, 110(7), pp. 956–957. Available at: https://doi.org/10.2105/AJPH.2020.305698

Lipsitch, M. (2020). 'Good Science is Good Science' in Thinking in a Pandemic: the Crisis of Science and Policy in the age of COVID-19. Cambridge: Verso Books. pp. 90–99.

Liu, C., Zhou, Q., Li, Y., Garner, L. V., Watkins, S. P., Carter, L. J., Smoot, J., Gregg, A. C., Daniels, A. D., Jervey, S. & Albaiu, D. (2020). Research and development on therapeutic agents and vaccines for COVID-19 and related human coronavirus diseases. *ACS Central Science*, 6(3), pp. 315 – 331. Available at: https://doi.org/10.1021/acscentsci.0c00272

Madeira, C. (2020). The impact of the COVID public policies on the Chilean households. *Applied Economics Letters*. 7th of October. Available at: https://doi.org/10.1080/13504851.2020.1832194

Majone, G. (2014). From regulatory state to a democratic default. *JCMS: Journal of Common Market Studies*, 52(6), pp. 1216 – 1223. Available at: https://doi.org/10.1111/jcms.12190

Mazey, S., & Richardson, J. (2020). Lesson-Drawing from New Zealand and Covid-19: The Need for Anticipatory Policy Making. *The Political Quarterly*, 91(3), pp. 561 – 570. Available at: https://doi.org/10.1111/1467-923X.12893

McCallum, M., Walls, A. C., Bowen, J. E., Corti, D. & Veesler, D. (2020). Structure-guided covalent stabilization of coronavirus spike glycoprotein trimers in the closed conformation, *Nature Structural & Molecular Biology*, 27(1) pp. 942 – 949. Available at: https://doi.org/10.1038/s41594-020-0483-8

McConnell, A. (2010). Policy success, policy failure and grey areas in-between. *Journal of Public Policy*, 30(3), pp. 345 – 362. Available at: https://doi.org/10.1017/S0143814X10000152

McKay, A. M., & Wozniak, A. (2020). Opaque: an empirical evaluation of lobbying transparency in the UK. *Interest Groups & Advocacy*, 9, pp. 102 – 118. Available at: https://doi.org/10.1057/s41309-019-00074-9

McKeever, A. (2020). "Coronavirus is Officially a Pandemic. Here's Why that Matters." *National Geographic*. 11th of March. Available at: https://www.nationalgeographic.com/science/article/how-coronavirus-could-become-pandemic-and-why-it-matters

McMillen, C.W. (2016). *Pandemics: A Very Short Introduction*. Oxford: Oxford University Press.

Mehellou, Y., Rattan, H. S., & Balzarini, J. (2017). The ProTide Prodrug Technology: From the Concept to the Clinic. *Journal of Medicinal Chemistry*, 61(6), pp. 2211 – 2226. Available at: https://doi.org/10.1021/acs.jmedchem.7b00734

Méndez, C. A. (2021). "The politics of the Covid-19 pandemic response in Chile" in Greer, S. L., King, E. J., Massard da Fonseca, E., & Perlata-Santos, A. (eds.) *Coronavirus politics: the comparative politics and policy of Covid-19*. Ann Arbor: University of Michigan Press, pp. 522 – 540.

Migone, A. R. (2020a). The influence of national policy characteristics on COVID-19 containment policies: a comparative analysis. *Policy Design and Practice*, 3(3), pp. 259 – 276. Available at: https://doi.org/10.1080/25741292.2020.1804660

Migone, A. R. (2020b). Trust, but customize: federalism's impact on the Canadian COVID-19 response. *Policy and Society*, 39(3), pp. 382 – 402. Available at: https://doi.org/10.1080/14494035.2020.1783788

Mintrom, M., & O'Connor, R. (2020). The importance of policy narrative: effective government responses to Covid-19. *Policy Design and Practice*, 3(3), pp. 205 – 227. Available at: https://doi.org/10.1080/25741292.2020.1813358

Monrad, J. T., Sandbrink, J. B., & Cherian, N. G. (2021). 'Promoting versatile vaccine development for emerging pandemics', *NPJ Vaccines*, 6(26), pp. 1 – 26. Available at: https://doi.org/10.1038/s41541-021-00290-y

Moon, S., Sridhar, D., Pate, M. A., Jha, A. K., Clinton, C., Delaunay, S., Edwin, V., Fallah, M., Fidler, D. P., Gerrett, L., Goosby, E., O Gostin, L., Heymann, D. L., Lee, K., Leung, G. M., Morrison, J. S., Saavedra, J., Tanner, M., Leigh, J. A., Hawkins, B., Woskie, L. R. & Piot, P. (2015). Will Ebola change the game? Ten essential reforms before the next pandemic. The report of the Harvard-LSHTM Independent Panel on the Global Response to Ebola. *The Lancet*, 386(10009), pp. 2204–2221. Available at: https://doi.org/10.1016/S0140-6736(15)00946-0

Offe, C., (2021). 'Corona Pandemic Policy' in G. Delanty (ed.), *Pandemics, Politics, and Society* (Berlin: De Gruyter), 25–41

Pandey, A., & Saxena, N. K. (2020). Effectiveness of Government Policies in Controlling COVID-19 in India. *International Journal of Health Services*. 29th of December. Available at: https://doi.org/10.1177%2F0020731420983749

Park, J. (2021). Who is hardest hit by a pandemic? Racial disparities in COVID-19 hardship in the US. *International Journal of Urban Sciences*, 25(2), pp. 149–177. Available at: https://doi.org/10.1080/12265934.2021.1877566

Parsell, C., Clarke, A., & Kuskoff, E. (2020). Understanding responses to homelessness during COVID-19: an examination of Australia. *Housing Studies*. 5th of October. Available at: https://doi.org/10.1080/02673037.2020.1829564

Paul, E., Steptoe, A., & Fancourt, D. (2021). Attitudes towards vaccines and intention to vaccinate against COVID-19: Implications for public health communications. *The Lancet Regional Health-Europe*, 1, p. 100012. Available at: https://doi.org/10.1016/j.lanepe.2020.100012

Phillips, S. (2006). Current status of surge research. *Academic Emergency Medicine*, 13(11), pp. 1103–1108. Available at: https://doi.org/10.1197/j.aem.2006.07.007

Plümper, T., & Neumayer, E. (2020). Lockdown policies and the dynamics of the first wave of the Sars-CoV-2 pandemic in Europe. *Journal of European Public Policy*. 27th of November. Available at: https://doi.org/10.1080/13501763.2020.1847170

Political and Constitutional Reform Committee (2013). *The Government's lobbying Bill.* Political and Constitutional Reform (7th report). London: The Stationery Office. Available at: www.parliament.uk/pcrc

Priori, R., Pellegrino, G., Colafrancesco, S., Alessandri, C., Ceccarelli, F., Di Franco, M., Riccieri, V., Scrivo, R., Sili Scavalli, A., Romana Spinelli, F. & Conti, F. (2021). SARS-CoV-2 vaccine hesitancy among patients with rheumatic and musculoskeletal diseases: a message for rheumatologists. *Annals of the Rheumatic Diseases,* 80(7), pp. 953–954. Available at: http://dx.doi.org/10.1136/annrheumdis-2021-220059

Pulla P. (2020). What counts as a covid-19 death? *BMJ*, 370(1), pp. 1–2. Available at: http://dx.doi.org/10.1136/bmj.m2859

Raj, M. (2021). "India's response to Covid-19" in Greer, S. L., King, E. J., Massard da Fonseca, E., & Perlata-Santos, A. (eds.) *Coronavirus politics: the comparative politics and policy of Covid-19.* Ann Arbor: University of Michigan Press, pp. 178–195.

Riedel, S. (2005). Edward Jenner and the history of smallpox and vaccination. *Proc (Bayl Univ Med Cent),* 18(1), pp. 21–25. Available at https://doi.org/10.1080/08998280.2005.11928028

Robert, A. (2020). Lessons from New Zealand's COVID-19 outbreak response. *The Lancet Public Health*, 5(11), pp. e569-e570. Available at: https://doi.org/10.1016/S2468-2667(20)30237-1

Ruger, J. P., & Yach, D. (2009). The global role of the World Health Organization. *Global Health Governance*, 2(2), pp. 1–11. Available at: https://www.ncbi.nlm.nih.gov/pmc/articles/PMC3981564/

Seccareccia, M. & Rochon, L. P. (2020). What Have We Learned from the COVID-19 Crisis? Domestic and International Dimensions and Policy Options for a Post-Coronavirus World: Introduction, *International Journal of Political Economy*, 49(4), pp. 261–264, Available at: https://doi.org/10.1080/08911916.2020.1857588

Serikbayeva, B., Abdulla, K., & Oskenbayev, Y. (2020). State capacity in responding to COVID-19. *International Journal of Public Administration*. 7th of December. Available at: https://doi.org/10.1080/01900692.2020.1850778

Shin, I., & Ju, S. T. (2020). Korean Government's response to COVID-19: role of Ministry of Food and Drug Safety (MFDS). *International Review of Public Administration*, 25(4), pp. 279–292. Available at: https://doi.org/10.1080/12294659.2020.1858585

Shiraki, K., & Daikoku, T. (2020). Favipiravir, an anti-influenza drug against life-threatening RNA virus infections. *Pharmacology & therapeutics*, 209(1), p. 107512. Available at: https://doi.org/10.1016/j.pharmthera.2020.107512

Singer, P. M., Willison, C. E., Moore-Petinak & N., Greer, S. L. (2021). "Anatomy of a failure: Covid-19 in the United States" in Greer, S. L., King, E. J., Massard da Fonseca, E., & Perlata-Santos, A. (eds.) *Coronavirus politics: the comparative politics and policy of Covid-19*. Ann Arbor: University of Michigan Press, pp. 478–493.

Sloan, S. M. (2020). Behind the 'Curve': COVID-19, Infodemic, and Oral History. *The Oral History Review*, 47(2), pp. 193–202. Available at: https://doi.org/10.1080/00940798.2020.1798256

Soremi, T., & Dogo, S. (2021). Gender and pandemic generals: analyzing policy response to COVID-19 in Ontario, Canada and Scotland, United Kingdom. *Policy Design and Practice*, 4(1), pp. 133–151. Available at: https://doi.org/10.1080/25741292.2020.1864120

Stylianou, V. (2021). A policy response to COVID-19: An Australian perspective. *Journal of the International Council for Small Business*. 18th of February. Available at: https://doi.org/10.1080/26437015.2020.1852060

Tortorici, M. A., Beltramello, M., Lempp, F. A., Pinto, D., Dang, H. V., Rosen, L. E., *et al.* (2020). Ultrapotent human antibodies protect against SARS-CoV-2 challenge via multiple mechanisms. *Science*, 370(6519), pp. 950–957. Available at: https://doi.org/10.1126/science.abe3354

Vera-Valdés, J. E. (2021). The political risk factors of COVID-19. *International Review of Applied Economics*, 35(2), pp. 269–287. Available at: https://doi.org/10.1080/02692171.2020.1866973

Walls, A. C. , Park, Y.-J., Tortorici, M. A., Wall, A., McGuire, A. T., & Veesler, D. (2020). Structure, function and antigenicity of the SARS-CoV-2 spike glycoprotein. *Cell*, 181(1), pp. 281–292.e1-e6. Available at: https://doi.org/10.1016/j.cell.2020.11.032

Weisblum, Y., Schmidt, F., Zhang, F., DaSilva, J., Poston, D., Lorenzi, J. C., Muecksch, F., Rutkowska, M., Hoffmann, H.-H., Michailidis, E., Gaebler, C., Agudelo, M., Cho, A., Wang, Z., Gazumyan, A., Cipolla, M., Luchsinger, L., Hillyer, C. D., Caskey, M., Robbiani, D. F., Rice, C. M., Nussenzweig, M. C., Hatziioannou, T., & Bieniasz, P. D. (2020). Escape from neutralizing antibodies by SARS-CoV-2 spike protein variants. *Elife*, 9(1), p. e61312. Available at: https://doi.org/10.7554/eLife.61312

White, K. M., Rosales, R., Yildiz, S., Kehrer, T., Miorin, L., Moreno, E., Jangra, S., Uccellini, M. B., Rathnasinghe,R., Coughlan, L., Martinez-Romero, C., Batra, J., Rojc, A., Bouhaddou, M., Fabius, J. M., Obernier, K., Dejosez, M., Guillén, M. J., Losada, A., Avilés, P., Schotsaert, M., Zwaka, T., Vignuzzi, M., Shokat, K. M., Krogan, N. J., & García-Sastre, A. (2021). Plitidepsin has potent preclinical efficacy against SARS-CoV-2 by targeting the host protein eEF1 A. *Science*, 371(6532), pp. 926–931. Available at: https://doi.org/10. 1126/science.abf4058

Wilson, D. B., Solomon, T. A., & McLane-Davison, D. (2020). Ethics and Racial Equity in Social Welfare Policy: Social Work's Response to the COVID-19 Pandemic. *Social Work in Public Health*, 35(7), pp. 617–632. Available at: https://doi.org/10.1080/19371918.2020. 1808145

Wood, J. G., Zamani, N., MacIntyre, C. R., & Beckert, N. G. (2007). Effects of internal border control on spread of pandemic influenza. *Emerging Infectious Diseases*, 13(7), pp. 1038–1045. Available at: https://doi.org/10.3201/eid1307.060740

WHO. (2018). *Managing Epidemics*. Geneva: World Health Organization. Available at: https:// www.who.int/emergencies/diseases/managing-epidemics-interactive.pdf

WHO. (2020). *WHO Director-General's Opening Remarks at the Media Briefing on COVID-19–11 March 2020*. Geneva: World Health Organization. Available at: https://www.who. int/dg/speeches/detail/who-directorgeneral-s-opening-remarks-at-the-media-briefing-on-covid-19-11-march-2020

WHO. (2021). *WHO-convened global study of origins of SARS-CoV-2: China part. Joint WHO-China study, 14 January-10 February 2021*. Geneva: WHO. Available at: https://www.who. int/publications/i/item/who-convened-global-study-of-origins-of-sars-cov-2-china-part

Yamey, G., Schäferhoff, M., Aars, O. K., Bloom, B., Carroll, D., Chawla, M., Dzau, V., Echalar, R., Singh Gill, I., Godal, T., Gupta, S., Jamison, D., Kelley, P., Kristensen, F., Mundaca-Shah, C., Oppenheim, B., Pavlin, J., Salvado, R., Sands, P., Schmunis, R., Soucat, A., Summers, L. H., El Turabi, A., Waldman, R. & Whiting, E. (2017). Financing of international collective action for epidemic and pandemic preparedness. *The Lancet Global Health*, 5(8), pp. e742-e744. Available at: https://doi.org/10.1016/S2214-109X(17) 30203-6

Yanzhong H (2009). Surge Response Capability and Pandemic Preparedness in *Pandemic Preparedness in Asia*, Caballero-Anthony, M. (ed.). Singapore: S. Rajaratnam School of International Studies. pp. 92–102. Available at: https://www.jstor.org/stable/re srep05905.18

Yiu, R. C., Yiu, C. P. B., & Li, V. Q. T. (2020). Evaluating the WHO's framing and crisis management strategy during the early stage of COVID-19 outbreak. *Policy Design and Practice*, 4(1), pp. 94–114. Available at: https://www.tandfonline.com/doi/full/10.1080/ 25741292.2020.1853337

Zhou, F., Yu, T., Du, R., Fan, G., Liu, Y., Liu, Z., Xiang, J., Wang, Y., Song, B., Gu X., Guan, L., Wei, Y., Li, H., Wu, X., Xu, J., Tu, S., Zhang, T., Chen, H., & Cao, B. (2020). Clinical course and risk factors for mortality of adult inpatients with COVID-19 in Wuhan, China: a retrospective cohort study. *The Lancet*, 395(10229), pp. 1054–1062. Available at: https:// doi.org/10.1016/S0140-6736(20)30566-3

Zhou, P., Yang, XL., Wang, XG. *et al.* (2020). A pneumonia outbreak associated with a new coronavirus of probable bat origin. *Nature*, 579, pp. 270–273. Available at: https://doi. org/10.1038/s41586-020-2012-7

www.ingramcontent.com/pod-product-compliance
Lightning Source LLC
Chambersburg PA
CBHW052012270326
41929CB00015B/2882